26 WAYS TO KEEP MOVING

The joyful connections people make
with their physical selves

Dr Gordon Spence & Riley Spence

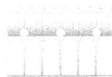

LONGUEVILLE
MEDIA

First published 2022 for Gordon Spence and Riley Spence by

LONGUEVILLE
MEDIA

Longueville Media Pty Ltd
PO Box 205
Haberfield NSW 2045 Australia
www.longmedia.com.au
info@longmedia.com.au

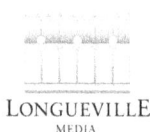

Artwork by Alison Zammit
Cover by Christabella Designs

The Health Activation Process is intellectual property and a trademark of MindTrek Coaching Services Pty Ltd and may only be used with permission. ALL RIGHTS RESERVED

ISBN: 978-0-6456150-2-9
ISBN POD: 978-0-6457109-6-0
ISBN eBook: 978-0-6457109-7-7

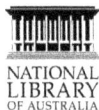

To Anita & Ella

For supporting this little obsession of ours.

With thanks to Marina, Neil, Oliver, Donna, Aimee, Eddie, Tyan, Ellie, Aylin, Shane, Kesley, Alex, Vinnie, Susan, Kristen, Matt, Alise, Zoe, Kristen, Pete, Craig, Deanne, Dickie, Melissa, Emma, and Kashi for generously agreeing to be part of this project and for sharing their experiences so openly. Thanks also to Picrina, who agreed to help put some icing on the cake!

Contents

Foreword

I first met Gordon and Riley a few years back at our local parkrun. I think Gordon beat me and I just beat Riley – but that's not relevant. What is relevant is that I always like to chat to those I run against. Invariably, I tell them about the group of runners that my husband, Robert, and I coach each week at the local athletic track. I tell them that we have a great social group, and that we offer a solid workout that will help them to run better and, hopefully, faster. When I spoke to Gordon and Riley that first time, I remember seeing a glint in Gordon's eye as he learned about a chance to hang out with others who also enjoyed running. Both were keen to become better runners and connect with a group that could keep them on track.

This is Gordon's second book in a career transformation that began over two decades ago. Looking for more job satisfaction, he took himself back to school at the age of 31 to become a psychologist, and, soon after, got married, became a lecturer, and started a family. In the process, the interest he had for running as a younger man went into hibernation and stayed that way for almost 20 years. When he turned 48, Gordon was looking for a little more out of life and so he started running again. This led to a physical transformation, and he was loving it! After setting some challenging goals and entering some events, he became so intrigued by what was happening that – at the age of 51 – he enrolled in an exercise science degree. This has led him to becoming an author and sharing his experience and knowledge with others.

In his first book, *Get Moving Keep Moving*, Gordon shared the joy and energy of his transformations. It's a great workbook for helping people find their way back to physical activity in an enjoyable way. In this second book, co-authored with his son Riley, they continue with that theme as they explore *26 Ways to Keep Moving*.

According to Google, there are over 800 recognised sports. Gordon and Riley have chosen a very interesting selection of physical pursuits and used the 26 letters of the alphabet to organise them. Starting with 'A' for alpine skiing, all the way through to 'Z' for zurkhaneh, they have chosen things designed to get you thinking. Possible options for starting your journey, something that will inspire you to get moving and keep moving.

For me, I've been fortunate to have had a consistent exercise regime from almost 50 years. I started exercising simply to keep my weight under control and over the years have played hockey, squash, tennis, and golf, and been a surfer too. I have also always loved running and set goals to compete in national and international competitions. My activity patterns and routines have always motivated me, and I started coaching so I could include some companions in my workouts. As I helped my athletes enjoy their journeys, the coaching keeps reminding me about the importance of goals and routines, as they provide the incentive to exercise regularly, especially when daily life tries to get in the way.

This book opens the door to an array of physical activity options that could build a platform for healthy ageing and bring considerable joy to your life. It showcases options that can be enjoyed alone, in pairs, in a team, or within a club. Some that require specialised equipment and some not at all. Some that have some cost or no cost. Within these pages I hope you'll find inspiration. The inspiration to go out and try something that appeals to you – something that might give you a wild ride, a rough ride, a smooth ride, or a slow ride. It doesn't have to be serious; it's just best if it's regular. Ideally, something that becomes part of your lifestyle.

So, enjoy the read and be bold. Engage your imagination and then transform it into reality!

Margaret Beardslee, OAM
Triathlon and Athletic Coach
Twice World Age Duathlon Champion

Preface

It's only a matter of months since *Get Moving Keep Moving: Healthy Ageing and How Physical Activity Loves You Back* was published. Clearly, this is the follow-up. But why so soon? After all, when you finish a book, the strong temptation is to say, 'Hallelujah, I'm done! Now, hand me a stiff drink, then I'm off for a good lie down.' However, I had a strong urge to start writing again. After several weeks promoting the book, doing a couple of launches, and blogging about its key themes, I felt I'd left something undone. Let me explain.

If you've read the first book, you'll recall that I introduced you to the Health Activation Process, a model with these four reflective stages:

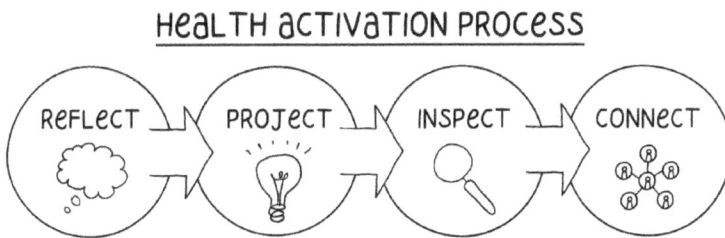

HeaLTH aCTIVaTION PROCeSS

REFLECT ▷ PROJECT ▷ INSPECT ▷ CONNECT

As you might also recall, I worked you through this model with the deliberate intention of not telling you what to do. I did this because an awful lot of public health promotion is prescriptive and geared towards telling people how to move, eat, drink, and sleep. But, deep down, most people don't like being told what to do. This wasn't a criticism of health promotion, mind you. Far from it. We need health promotion. People need to know about health issues and be given some guidance. The problem I see is that, for several health-related issues – diet, exercise, sleep – people have been told, and told, and told, and told. So much so, there's a risk people start to hear certain health messages as a form of white noise and tune them out. I wrote the first book because I thought there was another way to go about it, and *Get Moving Keep Moving* was the presentation of that other way.

My starting assumption for *Get Moving Keep Moving* was simply this: Human beings come into the world with an in-built love of physical activity. You probably loved it as a kid, and maybe an adolescent, and even in early adulthood, but along the way you might have lost that love, or at least got disconnected from it. After life went and got all busy on you, what was once essential effort soon became discretionary effort. To put it another way, your 'must have' may have become a 'nice to have'.

As such, the book was about reconnections with physical activity. The first step – REFLECT – plunged right in. It challenged you to remember back to your childhood and adolescence, to a time when physical activity may have been more central to your life, and to reminisce about those times. That was all about getting inside those early experiences and looking for what was positive and enjoyable. Then – in PROJECT – you were encouraged to use that as a basis to make some decisions about what you might like to do, moving forward.

And this is where I felt I missed an opportunity. In my keenness to keep the book compact and readable, too little time was spent helping readers explore potentially enjoyable forms of physical activity. Sure, I mentioned a few things – running got some attention, and so did rowing, cycling, and swimming, but beyond that, there wasn't very much. That's what this book is about: different ways to keep moving.

One of the things that's become super clear to me recently is that most of us live in communities that are jam-packed with different physical activity options. And within those communities are people who absolutely love what they do. Dedicated, devoted souls. People who live and breathe their chosen physical pursuit and, more than that, see it as essential scaffolding for their life. Something they simply cannot do without.

So, I wanted to explore that by talking to people who love their chosen physical pursuits. Present a showcase of different ways that people compete in sports or engage in active recreation. In my mind, it wasn't especially important what would be covered, so long as it was diverse and interesting. As such, I decided to opt for an A-to-Z arrangement, with *26 Ways to Keep Moving* the obvious title.

Now, we'd like to be clear about something. Like the first book, this book is not going to tell you what to do. None of the physical pursuits in this book is being presented with any sort of special endorsement or personal recommendation. All we are seeking to do is present a broad sample of the many options that exist. But more than that, we want you to hear from people who are devoted to their pursuits, to gain an insight into what they love about what they do, what thrills and excites them, what they find satisfying, and how it fills their life. In doing this, our hope is that you will have your horizons expanded, so you can think more creatively about what might be right for you.

The first thing to say about this book is that whilst the selection of physical pursuits is rather random, it is not completely random. On the one hand, we've allowed the alphabet to constrain our choices. So, because there's only one 'S' in the alphabet, we've only included one sport starting with 'S', knowing full well there are many more. In this case, we chose surfing, but it could just as easily have included swimming, shot put, soccer, softball, skateboarding, or sailing. Why surfing, and not one of the others? Our reasons for choosing the different pursuits vary a bit. Sometimes it was simply because we knew someone who loved that physical pursuit (e.g., surfing and mountain biking), or because it intrigued us (e.g., luge and fencing), or because we found it amusing (e.g., bog snorkelling and extreme ironing). On one occasion – 'Z' – it was a lack of other options. However, in the case of zurkhaneh, we welcomed this absence of choice, because it allowed us to focus on a little-known physical pursuit that has deep cultural and historical roots.

On the other hand, we did balance these choice limitations by making choices in other ways. For instance, the sport of swimming does get covered, under open-water swimming, and sailing gets included via yachting. Sure, we've taking some liberties with our classification, which might be cheating a bit but, hey, we're ok with that. Our aim is to present a cross section of different physical pursuits, and if playing with the labelling of a sport or physical pursuit helps us do that, no problem!

But our choices were also influenced by our interest in including physical pursuits that might not be considered mainstream. As a rule, we avoided higher profile activities, like cricket, rugby, soccer, tennis, golf, and basketball, as these have some of the highest community participation rates and get the most amount of the attention. Rather, we wanted to cast a much wider net, and try to balance some more conventional pursuits (e.g., netball, skiing, ice skating) with less conventional pursuits (e.g., bog snorkelling, quadball, vigoro). Within this collection, we hope you'll find some interest and some inspiration. We hope you'll start thinking about physical activity in ways you never have before, and view the possibilities surrounding you like you've never seen before – through a lens of deep enjoyment and satisfaction. Something you might feel inspired to go out and create for yourself.

As I found with *Get Moving Keep Moving*, solo authorship has many advantages and many disadvantages. Sure, you get to work at your own pace and have maximum creative control, but it can be a slow, painstaking, and lonesome business. As such, there's always a temptation to try writing with someone else. And if you find the right person, it can be an absolute joy.

When I had the idea for a follow-up book, I thought the structure suited a writing collaboration. By choosing to highlight

26 different physical pursuits and using a consistent chapter structure (i.e., description, origins, rules, personal story), the work could be broken up into distinct chunks, worked on separately, and then combined into a whole. That seemed like a good approach and one that might also be fun, depending on the person.

For me, the obvious person was my 15-year-old son, Riley. There were a few reasons for this. First, he has a natural interest in sport and physical activity. Second, the book needed someone who knows how to research, and that's a skill he's been developing throughout high school. Third, for the sake of my sanity, I wanted someone who would be easy to work with, and he's always been that. And, finally, the book needed someone who could write. Whilst Riley has developed into a decent writer, he hasn't always enjoyed writing. He'd found it a bit dull, and boring. And so, I wondered, what if he got involved in a writing project on a topic of real interest? Would he develop a different perspective on it and possibly even enjoy it? Maybe. In any case, it seemed like an idea that was worth running by him – so I did. Once I'd explained the idea, his response was immediate. He liked the idea and was up for the challenge.

The very next day, the Spence & Son writing collaboration began its work.

And now a word from the Researcher-in-Chief…

If someone had told me before this year I'd be co-authoring a book when I was 15, I would've laughed in their face and complimented them on their sense of humour. Ever since I stepped foot into my kindergarten English class with Mrs Bellwood, I've never been thrilled about doing any sort of writing. That wasn't my teacher's fault – I just felt it was rather boring and a waste of my time. My views on writing didn't really change all that much until about Year 9. This was the first year I didn't moan and complain when I checked my timetable and saw I had an English class. Kudos to

Mr Andrew, my English teacher, for that. Luckily, he is still my teacher this year. Throughout the last year and a half in his class, I've realised that writing doesn't kill you. Eureka! Cheers, sir!

So, when Dad asked me about writing this book with him, I thought I'd take him up on the offer. I figured that by writing about something that really interests me, it might be possible to get some enjoyment out of it. I have a big interest in sport and physical activity, so I knew that spending time researching different physical pursuits, interviewing people who did them, and then writing about it probably wouldn't be a chore or a hardship for me. As it turns out, it wasn't a hardship, and it was kind of fun.

We hope you enjoy it!

An A-to-Z Guide of Physical Pursuits

A short note before you start

When we started writing this book, we felt it was probably not the type of book that people would read cover to cover, in three or four sittings. Being a book of 26 stories, we felt it might be more like a coffee table book – a book people might pick up, scan the table of contents for something interesting, read a chapter or two, and then put it down again until the next day. Obviously, people can decide for themselves how they want to read it. That's just how it felt to us.

As you read, we hope you might be inspired enough to go out and try one of the 26 Ways to Keep Moving, or do something else that's come to mind. If you do feel so inspired, you may also be keen to know a little more. So, to help with that, we are supporting these stories with the following:

A gallery of photos, provided by the contributors, so that you can see them all in action.

Internet links to the various sport and recreation bodies (clubs, associations, governing bodies) that will give you a way to find local contacts and get involved, should you wish to.

To access the photo gallery and internet links, please scan the QR codes over the page. They will take you to www.healthyageingproject.com, where the photos and links are continuously updated.

Use this QR code find out how to connect with various clubs, associations or businesses involved with the 26 Ways.

Use this QR code to view a photo gallery of the 26 Ways contributors and their chosen physical pursuits.

Alpine Skiing

What is it?

It may be stating the obvious, but skiing is the action of gliding over snow using long, flat runners – skis – attached to specially designed boots. Whilst skiing is still used in some parts of the world as a basic and vital form of transportation, it is more commonly recognised as a sport that people participate in competitively or recreationally. We should note here that alpine skiing is the traditional name for what is also known as downhill skiing, or simply 'downhill', a competitive form of the sport best known from the Winter Olympics. But this chapter isn't about competitive downhill racing; it's about the non-competitive recreational pursuit enjoyed by many millions of people worldwide.

Whilst skiing has three main types – alpine, Nordic (cross-country and ski jumping), and telemark – multiple variations have developed over the years. These include snowboarding, skiboarding, and several freestyle skiing variations, such as moguls, aerials, ski cross, half-pipe, and slopestyle. Based on the evolution of the sport, it would appear human beings greatly enjoy gliding over snow! Given that the Winter Olympics program currently includes up to 10 skiing variations, that's a reasonable conclusion.

What are its origins?

Skiing is a sport with an ancient past and represents an adaptation of human beings to living in cold climates. The earliest indications of ski-like objects have been found in northern Russia and date back to around 7,000 BC. Other evidence includes depictions of skiing in 4,000-year-old Norwegian rock carvings, and fragments of skis preserved in Scandinavian bogs (circa 1,500 BC to 1,000 AD). It appears that the earliest skis were short and broad, something more akin to snowshoes, and not the narrow runners we're used to seeing today. Aside from basic transportation, skiing was widely used for hunting, especially by the Samis and other peoples of Scandinavia and Russia. It has also been used for military purposes as far back as the 13th century, and as recently as World War II.

As a sport, skiing started to gain popularity in the 19th century, with the first cross-country, downhill, and ski-jumping competitions being held in Norway and North America during the mid-1800s. As a recreational pursuit, the popularity of skiing was enhanced by several important equipment innovations, most notably with boots and bindings, but was most dramatically influenced by the invention of the ski lift in the 1930s. This meant that skiers no longer needed to complete exhausting mountain ascents before they could ski, and could manage multiple runs in a day, rather than just a few. This gave the sport a much broader appeal and helped to increase its popularity, so much so that alpine skiing was included in the Winter Olympics program at the 1936 Garmisch-Partenkirchen games in Germany. After the arrival of broadcast television in the 1950s, images of skiing were screened around the world, further popularising the sport and establishing it as a major focal point of any Winter Olympics.

What rules, if any, does it have?

Given this chapter is focused more on recreational skiing than competitive skiing, a description of its rules makes little sense. Perhaps the only rules we can point to are moral rules – rules related to acting responsibly and respectfully when swooshing down the slopes. After all, skiing is not without its risks, and if people behave recklessly on a busy ski run, they won't just endanger themselves. Whilst being responsible can mean giving way to people and taking turns, it can also mean skiing only on slopes you're skilled enough to cope with, and not in areas where specialised knowledge or training might be required. After all, if you get too ambitious and wrap yourself around a tree, or get caught in a blizzard, away from help, you'll have to rely on someone else to make things right.

The joy of it all

Marina is a 51-year-old coaching psychologist. She's been skiing since she was five and has never missed a season in all that time. For her, skiing is just what you do when winter arrives. This was instilled in her from an early age, by parents who met on the ski field at Mt Hotham in Victoria and went on to share their love of adventuring with Marina and her three older siblings. In her family, one's fifth birthday was quite a big deal. That's because it was the age you were allowed to go to the ski lodge. Back then, Mt Hotham was not well enough developed to cater for very young children. So, becoming 'a big girl' had a special significance for her. It unlocked the door to a world that she immediately loved and has continued to love ever since. Skiing has been one of the constants in her life, perhaps even *the* constant.

The most fun you can have on two legs

As a sport, skiing carries many positive memories for Marina. One of the earliest was the special memory of simply being grown up enough to join her family on the slopes, and the exhilarating feeling of travelling fast down a mountain. She vividly remembers what it was like being that young girl, full of energy and barrelling down the slopes with the exuberance of youth. But for her, skiing also got its sense of awesomeness from its connection to family holidays, and a strong feeling of freedom that she values to this day. From what we know of other skiers, this is not an uncommon feeling.

Having been introduced to skiing at a relatively early age, Marina got quite good at it, so much so that she skied competitively during her university years. But the sport's competitive possibilities were never a driving force for her. She was more motivated by a love of mountain country and the opportunities it gave her to go adventuring. And 'adventuring' is the appropriate word for Marina. When pressed about how she would rank skiing against other forms of physical activity, there was no hesitation: skiing is her favourite. Except then she did hesitate, took a moment, and modified her answer – to ski mountaineering!

Mountaineering with skis

Given the choice, Marina would choose ski mountaineering over anything else. As the name suggests, this involves climbing snow-covered mountains – with crampons, ice picks, and ropes – getting to the top (or close to it) and skiing back down. But not back down via well-groomed ski runs. Far from it! This form of skiing involves finding your own pathway down a mountain, which might include jumping ledges, avoiding crevices, and/or slaloming your way through a forest. It's a challenging type of skiing that's unpredictable and requires good improvisation, a type of skiing that enables her to access areas of high mountain country not possible with conventional skiing, something that really appeals to the adventurous side of her personality. However, when Marina became a parent, she quickly realised that ski mountaineering came with risks that she just couldn't justify. So, she made the decision to stop and switched her focus to teaching her kids to ski, so they could enjoy the sport together, as a family.

Telemark

Having made the responsible choice to put family skiing ahead of adventure skiing, Marina found herself a middle ground: telemark skiing. This is a form of skiing developed in Norway that combines alpine and cross-country skiing. How is this a middle ground? Simple. Telemark skiing uses boots and ski bindings that permit skiers to go up hills, whereas alpine skiers can only go down. So, for someone who likes a bit of mountain roaming, telemark is a great option. It's also an option that comes with an increased physical challenge, as the technique involves a repetitive lunging motion that gives one's quadricep muscles a decent workout.

Skiing this way gives Marina options whenever she hits the slopes. On the one hand she can use conventional gear to ski with her family and friends on resort runs. But she can also go 'off-piste' from time to time, get away from the busyness of a resort, and enjoy the serenity of less-visited areas of mountain back country. Best of all, she can do that without taking too much risk. So, telemarking really works for her, and has been a great source of enjoyment.

Skiing is like an onion

Whilst chatting about her love of skiing, Marina found it difficult to pinpoint the thing she liked the most about it. For her, skiing is like an onion – it has layers. Layers that include significant childhood memories, feelings of freedom, adrenaline hits, possibilities for adventure, connections with nature, and the chance to enjoy all that with family and friends. Any physical activity capable of delivering that much to your life is clearly worth a great deal. And that's probably just as well, because skiing isn't cheap. All the gear, all the travel, all the accommodation, etc., can really add up. At times, Marina pulls back and thinks the whole thing's a bit crazy, spending a bunch of money to take a chairlift to the top of a mountain, only to turn around and ski straight back down. However, there's no doubt in her mind that the investment is worth it. For her, skiing is an uplifting experience of the very best kind, something she can't imagine being without.

However, as much as she loves skiing, Marina is not an evangelist for it. She's never been the sort to try and convince others they should be doing it too. For one, she's sensitive to the fact that it's not within everyone's reach, financially or geographically. Aside from the equipment costs, skiing in Australia only happens in one small corner of the country, which means that it takes more planning and time to access than it does in more mountainous northern hemisphere countries. But Marina's life has allowed her to do it on a regular basis, and this is something that she's always been extremely grateful for.

Sharing the experience with others

Having said that, Marina has found ways to share her joy of skiing and mountain adventuring with others. One has been through her involvement with Outward Bound and leading mountain survival courses. These courses have allowed her to enjoy alpine environments in another way, by teaching people how to snow camp, where to set up tents, and what to be thinking about when moving around in high country areas. She's been able to do this because skiing brings sport and nature together in an intimate way. Unlike running or swimming, where you can engage with nature in a relatively comfortable way, skiing environments are much more hostile and unpredictable. So, when you go into alpine country, you need to know what you're doing. And Marina does. She knows how to measure snow depths and density, she knows about snow drifts, how snow moves around a mountain and where it builds up. Crucially, she knows how to detect the signs of avalanche and take the precautions needed to stay safe. You could say she's developed a form of 'natural intelligence' – a nuanced understanding of nature – that she feels compelled to share.

So, Marina has derived much from a life of skiing. It's a pursuit she has a deep affection for – even when the weather is 'filthy' and a chair by the fire seems like a better place to be. But there's just something about it, something that gets into your blood, and is hard to put words around. Something that's worth going back for, year after year.

Bog Snorkelling

What is it?

Bog snorkelling is a sport that involves propelling one's body through a 60-yard (55-metre) water-filled trench that's been cut through a peat bog. As it involves submersing oneself in bog water, competitors wear snorkels, diving masks, flippers, and more often than not, wetsuits. Whilst the sport has had a World Championship event since it started in 1985, few people take it too seriously. Nonetheless, competitors have been known to dedicate some focused effort to the sport, and world records are kept and updated each year. The current world records for covering a standard 120-yard (110-metre) course are one minute, 18 seconds for men, and one minute, 22 seconds for women. Both the current world record holders are English.

In recent years, bog snorkelling has developed some variants. These include mountain bike bog snorkelling, where the standard course is attempted on specially modified bikes weighted down with lead shot, and bog snorkelling triathlon, which combines the standard snorkelling distance with a 13-mile bike ride and an 8-mile run. Like conventional bog snorkelling, these alternatives are conducted within an atmosphere of extreme light-heartedness and considerable good humour.

What are its origins?

According to the BBC, bog snorkelling was created in Wales, in 1976. According to local folklore, it emerged from a discussion between regulars in a pub, around 50 km north of Cardiff. As a result, Wales is the spiritual home of bog snorkelling, and the World Championships take place every year there, in early spring, not far from that pub. Whilst some events have been run outside Wales, such as Julia Creek in north-west Queensland, nothing has yet come close to replacing Wales as the centre of the bog snorkelling world.

As such, the annual World Championship event in Llanwrtyd Wells gets, by far, the most attention, including regular coverage by the media. Such is the interest in bog snorkelling that the event effectively doubles as a summer community festival and has become an attraction for not just local people but visitors from nearby England, Ireland, and Scotland, and from the more distant Sweden, Japan, New Zealand, Australia, South Korea, and Russia. In a way that's consistent with the eccentric nature of the sport, competitors and visitors often compete and attend in fancy dress, such as mermaid costumes, and then spend the day enjoying a variety of locally produced food, beverages, arts, and crafts.

What rules, if any, does it have?

The rules of bog snorkelling are relatively straightforward. They include the following:

- The trench must be relatively straight and measure a total of 60 yards (55 metres) in length
- Competitors must complete two lengths of the trench in the shortest possible time
- The course must be completed without using conventional swimming strokes, although a form of dog paddle is permitted
- Competitors use their legs to propel themselves, assisted by flippers

The joy of it all

Neil is a 38-year-old art teacher who lives in south-west England, near Bath. He also just happens to hold the current bog snorkelling world record, one minute, 18 seconds, and is a four-time world champion, having won at the 2017, 2018, 2019 and 2022 events. Whilst this is all some considerable claim to fame, it's also a matter of some amusement to Neil. You see, he's only ever swum in a bog trench on four occasions. Four swims, four wins, four World Championships! Clearly, the guy was born for the sport.

It would be misleading of us to claim that Neil lives for the sport of bog snorkelling. He doesn't. His sport of choice is cycling, which is something he trains for and frequently competes at. Although he didn't know it the first time he snorkelled, the leg strength of a cyclist is quite an advantage when you're scuttling along the bottom of a bog trench. As he would find out, this gave him an important point of difference on race day.

Just something that had to be done

Neil found out about bog snorkelling long before he ever tried it. He first became aware of it through one of those general interest news stories that often cap the end of the television news. When he and some of his mates saw it, they were amused and immediately declared, 'We're doing that!'

Whilst it took them a few years to get around to it, get around to it they most certainly did. In late August 2017, Neil and his friends headed to the home of bog snorkelling, Llanwrtyd Wells in Central Wales, to give it a try. Around 170 competitors took part that year. Whilst that sounds like a lot, Neil quickly clarified that roughly half the field were wearing mermaid costumes or other humorous attire. For anyone with any sort of competitive instinct, this was reassuring because, as you submerge yourself in the trench, you know your chances of posting a good time are better than average.

And, so it was for Neil. His 2017 bog snorkelling debut went well and he registered a decent time. Then, like everyone else, he dried himself off and stood back to marvel at the sights and sounds of this truly unique event. As the day wore on, his time proved to be more than decent. So decent, in fact, that no one could better it and Neil sloshed his way off the bog that day a very surprised world champion.

Dealing with the pressure of success

After winning his first event, Neil was keen to defend his crown. But did that mean he felt the weight of expectation? Did he feel pressure to prove it wasn't a fluke? No, not at all. Sure, he was curious to see if he could post a quicker time, but that's natural enough for someone who enjoys competition. When the 2018 event rolled around, he got his answer. Not only did he win it again, but he set a world record in the process – an eight-second improvement on his 2017 effort. When he came back in 2019, he won for a third time, despite swallowing a fair bit of bog water at the 75-metre mark.

The thing you need to appreciate about bog snorkelling is that there's no real training or formal preparation for it. No internet gurus to consult, no books to read, no snorkelling squads to join. If you want to excel at this sport, then you have to do it with whatever raw talent you possess and a base of fitness you've acquired elsewhere. Given all that, it's fair to ask: Why include it in this book?

The love of bog snorkelling

To be honest, we're not clear it's possible to develop a love of bog snorkelling. Think about it – there you are, slopping around in the middle of Wales, in cold bog water with zero visibility, sharing a shallow trench with a multitude of bugs, a few small eels, and some frogs. Whatever way you frame it, that's a million miles from swooshing through fluffy spring snow on the slopes of a mountain.

However, after speaking to Neil, we think it's possible to develop an *affection* for bog snorkelling. The way he explained it, if you really want to go for it, there's a substantial physical challenge that comes with leg-powering your way through 110 metres of watery trench. And that's something that appeals to him.

Whilst most physical pursuits offer the opportunity for physical exertion, bog snorkelling offers something extra. It comes with a tinge of the ridiculous and a chance to celebrate, let's call it, one's inner-loony. This makes any bog snorkelling event a joyous affair, with people coming together for no other reason, really, than having a good laugh. To be more precise, what we're talking about qualifies as *Type II* fun – experiences that are miserable in the moment but fun in retrospect. Something you're happy to be over and done with, yet you revel in later, when you trade stories with others and appreciate the silliness of it all.

It offers something cycling and swimming do not

Now, as Neil rightly pointed out, bog snorkelling is not the only eccentric fringe sport out there. Cheese rolling, wife carrying and woolsack racing are all physical pursuits that come with a touch of the absurd. And he's tried a few, including husband dragging. But, so far, none have offered quite as much enjoyment as bog snorkelling. For him, there just seems to be something about the blend of physical challenge and lunacy that keeps him coming back.

As he explained, after spending years surrounded by the seriousness of competitive cycling and swimming, Neil finds the relaxed informality that exists along the banks of a bog trench a pleasing place to be. So he intends to keep going, and after a two-year event hiatus due to COVID-19, he's looking forward to the 2022 World Championships. Does he expect to win again? No idea. What he's more curious about is how fast is it possible to go. Whilst he's sure the record can be broken, he's also pretty sure that, at some stage, someone fitter and stronger than he will come along and record a faster time. When that day comes, Neil will be as pleased as anyone. And it won't stop him from re-entering, because winning has never been the driving force for him.

What a way to Keep Moving!

Clearly bog snorkelling is a 'sometimes sport'. As Neil told us, people only really do it a few times a year, and in only a few locations. As far as he's aware, no one ever trains specifically for it, although he has heard whispers of a small group in Wales that may have started snorkelling more regularly.

We think it's clear that bog snorkelling doesn't stand out as an obvious option to help you to get yourself moving. But we think it does stand out as an interesting (read: slight nutty) option if you're already moving and would like to test your fitness in a strange and unusual setting. You know, doing it just because you can. Adding some texture to your life, using Type II fun to make memories, to meet new and, no doubt, interesting people…

Finally, and we think this last point is crucial: The fun factor in bog snorkelling only exists because it happens in the presence of other people. As a solo sport, we reckon it'd be a bit dismal; Type II fun without the enjoyable 'after taste' – and no, we're not referring to the taste of bog water. Of course, we might be wrong about that, but that's our hunch.

So, there you have it – bog snorkelling, for your consideration and possible inclusion on your physical activity bucket list!

CrossFit

What is it?

CrossFit is a distinctly modern sport. It is a strength and conditioning approach made up of functional movements performed at high intensity. This means the exercises closely reflect everyday movements, like pushing, pulling, lunging, and squatting, which involve multiple joints and multiple muscle groups. The elements of a CrossFit class can include interval training, Olympic-style weightlifting, plyometrics, gymnastics, kettlebell swinging, and calisthenics. It is believed the approach develops better general fitness than more narrowly focused, specialised training (that focus on single muscle groups) and helps prepare people for the unexpected physical challenges they might encounter in life.

The name CrossFit refers to more than the sport. It also refers to a trademarked fitness system that has been sold under licence to an estimated 15,000 gyms in 162 countries around the world. A defining feature of these gyms is their Workout of the Day. This is an announcement made to the members of a gym and typically comprises a small set of exercises that are to be completed and repeated, as many times as possible, in a short period of time. To support motivation, these workouts are often scored to encourage competition and help track individual progress.

What are its origins?

CrossFit first emerged as a physical fitness approach in 2001. It was founded by two fitness trainers, Greg Glassman and Lauren Jenai, who opened a gym in Santa Cruz, California, and started posting their workouts online for clients. Due to the cross-disciplinary nature of these workouts, they quickly captured the interest of military personnel, police, and firefighters, and then, shortly after, other gyms began showing an interest in using the new workouts. Although the interest was initially modest, with only 13 affiliated gyms in 2005, its popularity grew very quickly, and by 2013, approximately 8,000 gyms had become licenced to run CrossFit workouts.

One of the reasons for the rapid global expansion of CrossFit was the emergence of the CrossFit Games. Established in 2007, the games started out as a 'Woodstock of Fitness', with a rather informal, social event held at a California ranch. Athletes competed in a range of events and accumulated points, with the best combined individual and group scorers crowned as winners. As word spread and its popularity increased, bigger venues had to be found, and qualification events were eventually added. Whilst the CrossFit Games have become a significant commercial event, these games have also given serious athletes a legitimate competitive focus, helped to build CrossFit's global brand, and established it as an exciting spectator sport.

What rules, if any, does it have?

In competitive CrossFit, points are accumulated over several exercise rounds, and are awarded based on where athletes finish, relative to others. So, in any round, whoever completes the most repetitions is the winner and gets 100 points, with points for other athletes awarded on a sliding scale that links to their finishing position (second place = 99 points, and so on). However, in CrossFit, the focus is on speed *and* accuracy. This means that good technique matters. So, scores are only validated if an athlete's pistol squats, burpees, kettlebell swings, and/or deadlifts are judged to have been performed correctly. Aside from its competition rules, there is also an etiquette that exists at CrossFit gyms. This includes basic health and safety rules, such as maintaining good hygiene on the gym floor, and using and storing equipment properly. In addition, it is expected that CrossFitters will always be respectful of others, encourage new-comers, and cultivate a positive gym culture.

The joy of it all

Oliver is 21 years old. He's a full-time exercise and sports science student and part-time CrossFit coach. For him, this is a great combination. At university he learns about exercise physiology, functional anatomy, biomechanics, and exercise prescription, and then, when coaching in the gym, he can immediately apply this knowledge. This is something he sees as important. As Oliver well knows, CrossFit doesn't have a great reputation. Whilst he's aware of the injury and health concerns that surround the sport, his personal experience of CrossFit has always been positive, and he's seen the benefit it can provide to others. As such, he views his degree as a way of making a positive contribution to the sport, by raising his own coaching standards and making it safer and more effective and enjoyable for clients.

'What the hell am I doing here?'

Oliver's life got off to a rough start. He was born with arterial septum defects, a congenital heart problem that required open heart surgery when he was six months old. Whilst the operation was a success, he also had some hormone issues throughout his childhood, which required regular visits to an endocrinologist until he was 18. Despite this, Oliver was as active as other kids his age, involved in swimming, Little Athletics, and surf lifesaving, and played cricket, soccer, and his preferred sport, rugby union.

Whilst he played rugby between the ages of seven and 15, by the time Oliver reached adolescence, he wasn't in great shape. He was still playing rugby, but he'd put on some weight and was physically struggling to get through the games. As part of an attempt to do something about it, his dad had been looking into some training options and suggested he visit the local CrossFit gym. Soon after, he found himself standing in that gym, surrounded by some incredibly fit people, feeling rather tubby and asking himself, 'What the hell am I doing here?'

A shock to the system

The first time Oliver when to CrossFit, he was looking for a general improvement in his level of conditioning, so that he could play some better rugby. As it happened, the gym was run by one of the best CrossFitters in Australia, a guy who had recently won the CrossFit regionals and has an incredible physique. He also happened to be a nice guy, very welcoming and super encouraging.

Although Oliver didn't really know what he'd be doing in that first workout, he had watched a few CrossFit training videos. Based on that, he expected he'd probably be doing lots of back squats, powerlifts, lunges, and similar exercises. He was wrong. Very wrong. What he got was lots of cardio – 30 minutes of continuous rowing and running intervals. It was a tubby, out-of-shape 15-year-old's worst nightmare, so much so that he seriously considered faking an injury and pulling out of the class. But he kept going, got himself through it, and ended up flat on his back, heaving with exhaustion.

More Type II fun

As Oliver would come to learn, ending up flat on your back is a common experience for CrossFitters. Paradoxically, it's also one of its great attractions. Even though he didn't enjoy that first session very much, he couldn't wait to go back. One of the reasons was that he found it quite humbling. It showed him just how much physical condition he lacked, and how much it might be possible to gain. Two days later, he was back for more, and soon after that, he was hooked.

Oliver describes CrossFit as having strongly addictive qualities, qualities that, he admits, would not appeal to everyone. But he loves it because he loves a challenge, and it never gets easier. CrossFit has a way of 'keeping things real' for him, because no matter how good he thinks he's getting, the next session will invariably be as challenging as the last. This leaves him feeling like there's no obvious upper limit to his level of fitness, and that it's possible to keep getting better. But that doesn't mean he loves everything about the training. He doesn't. It's just not possible. Why? Because when people push themselves to their physical limits, it tends to hurt quite a lot. But, as we just learned with bog snorkelling, enjoyment doesn't always have to occur in the moment. It can come later, when the effort is over, and the discomfort has faded. CrossFit seems a lot like that, another form of Type II fun.

From athlete to coach

Oliver's great enthusiasm for CrossFit eventually motivated him to become a coach. This happened when he was 18, two years after he stopped playing rugby, and a year after recovering from shoulder surgery. At this point, CrossFit had become his main form of physical activity. He had developed a regular training routine, and whilst he was taking part in some local events, he was doing it more for the fun than the competition. Significantly, Oliver was also starting to see that he had a real passion for strength and conditioning, and so he wanted to get more involved.

He started by doing the CrossFit Level 1 certificate course. This allowed him to start coaching and to earn a little money, but Oliver found he wanted to learn more about physical conditioning – a lot more. So, driven by his interests in human performance, injury prevention, and physical rehabilitation, he enrolled in a university degree and is using that to make an impact, one reflected in his basic coaching, which is to help clients (i) have the best hour of their day, (ii) improve their capacity or skill by at least 1%, and (iii) do it in a safe and effective way.

Happiest hour of the day

Whether thinking about it as an athlete or a coach, Oliver loves that CrossFit creates feelings of enjoyment and satisfaction by getting people to explore their physical capacities. He loves that it exists within a 'can do' culture, with people who are encouraging and supportive. It's something he enjoys being part of, both an athlete and a coach. But it's through coaching that he can exert the most influence, by interacting with clients in ways that help him to 'read the room' and run classes that work well for everyone.

He also likes that CrossFit self-selects clients based on personality, rather than physicality. This means that whilst not everyone is a natural athlete, they all come with a desire to improve and get better. It's a mindset Oliver says makes them relatively easy to train, because they are prepared to listen and take instruction. This is especially the case with his early morning groups, classes made up busy working adults, aged 30 to 45, who come looking for 'mental relief' at 5 am every day. He's heard it described as the 'happiest hour of the day', a time when clients can put the hassles and concerns of life on hold and fully embrace an entirely different sort of challenge.

Doing his bit

Despite all the negative attention that CrossFit has had, Oliver firmly believes in its value and potential. He knows it can be done safely, having experienced that himself and seen it in others.

He also knows a big part of the problem lies with its delivery and the impression that CrossFit is only what's seen in the big international competitions, with outrageous-looking workouts and hyped-up performances. It's an impression he believes sends athletes and coaches on unhelpful ego trips, putting themselves and others at unnecessary risk. For Oliver, CrossFit is a safe and effective form of physical activity – provided it's delivered well. And that's something he's all about. Doing it right, winding up flat on your back (of course!), and waiting for the fun to arrive.

Dragon Boating

What is it?

Dragon boat racing is a sport that involves high intensity paddling. Like competitive rowing, kayaking and canoeing, the aim is to travel a set distance in the fastest possible time, yet there are some substantial differences. First, dragon boats are substantially longer than conventional rowing 'shells', kayaks and canoes as they can seat up to 20 paddlers, a steerer, and a drummer who sets the stroke rate of the team. By comparison, the largest rowing crew has eight members, plus a coxswain who steers the boat. Second, dragon boats are heavier than other racing craft and, similar to Polynesian outriggers, they sit a bit higher out of the water. Finally, and more obviously, dragon boats are decorated in a way that reflects the Chinese origin of the sport. Not only are they equipped with a drum, usually made of water buffalo hide and wood, but they are also rigged with decorative Chinese dragon heads and tails.

At competitive regattas, dragon boat crews race over a variety of distances, the shortest being 200 metres and the longest being 2,000 metres. Longer races are known, some stretching up to eight and 16 km. One reason the sport is so popular is that it also caters for athletes of all ages. Events are organised for juniors upwards, including Premiers (under 30s), and 40s, 50s, and 60s age divisions.

What are its origins?

Dragon boating is a sport with ancient origins. Dragon boats have been used for racing in southern-central China for over 2,500 years. Some of the earliest races were organised in honour of the late warrior poet Qu Yuan, a Chinese politician and patriot who drowned himself in protest against the political corruption of his day. Legend has it the local people who admired him raced out onto the river in boats to retrieve his body but, when unable to do so, they dropped balls of sticky rice into the river so the fish would eat them instead of Qu Yuan's body.

In the centuries that followed, dragon boat festivals were held to commemorate the day of his death, a custom that became widespread. In time, dragon boating developed to become a keenly contested competitive sport and led to the 1991 establishment of the International Dragon Boat Federation (IDBF). In the 30-plus years since its formation, IDBF associations or federations have emerged in 89 countries and territories around the world. By any measure, this makes dragon boating a truly international sport.

What rules, if any, does it have?

Dragon boat races are quite frenetic. When you have half a dozen or more 22-person crews paddling furiously down the same stretch of water, some rules and regulations are needed. Some of those include:

- The use of boats is provided by the regatta organisers, with paddlers bringing their paddles and life vests. Not only does this keep the racing fair, but it means that teams do not need to transport large dragon boats to race venues.
- The use of shared equipment means that teams have an obligation to return equipment to organisers, intact and in a timely way.

- All paddlers must remain seated during a race, even if they drop their paddle.
- Penalties can be imposed on a crew by the organisers for violating any of the above rules or other safety procedures, or engaging in any behaviour that is not sportsperson-like.

The joy of it all

Donna is 54-year-old teacher's aide who works with neurodiverse children. She's also very keen on the sport of dragon boating. In fact, she loves it, so much so that she gave up playing netball – which she played and loved for 25 years – to give more focus to her paddling. But that's what Donna is like. She takes her team sports seriously and believes it's important to follow through on the commitments you make to a team. Not surprisingly, this ethic has seen her not only join as a crew member at her local club but also take on the role of club President.

Swapped a ball for a boat

As mentioned, Donna was a keen netballer for over two decades. Whilst this was a sport she greatly enjoyed, she doesn't play it anymore. Interestingly, that's not because she fell out of love with it. She didn't. Rather, her transition from netball and towards dragon boating happened through a strange twist of fate.

In 2017, Donna's netball team was competing at the World Masters Games in Auckland, New Zealand. During the tournament they found out that the next games, to be held in Japan, weren't including netball in the program. Left without an option to participate, Donna and her teammates wondered if there were another sport they might take up. As they were contemplating this, they bumped into a crew of dragon boaters and began asking them questions. The answers were enough to trigger their interest.

Six months later, at the age of 49, Donna went along to a give-it-a-go day at a local club. She loved it immediately. She liked the contrast to netball. She liked that it challenged her in a completely different way, the need to maintain upper body strength, to remain still and stable in the boat, the different demands on her endurance, and the experience of being part of a much larger team. It seemed like she was onto something.

Life is all about choices

Simultaneously enjoying two sports is a nice position to be in, and from 2017 onwards, that's exactly where Donna found herself. For the first couple of years, she ran the sports side by side, playing netball during the winter, and switching to dragon boating in the summer. This went well for a while, but as she got more into dragon boating, she found it harder to do justice to both. So, rather than frustrate herself by partially committing to the two, she made the hard decision and stopped playing netball.

Having committed to dragon boating, Donna went all in. She involved herself in the running of the club and eventually became its President. She was loving the sport, and the environment that surrounds it. The great thing was that the sport was giving back to her as much as she was giving to it. How exactly? Well, for one thing, with championship medals.

Standing on a podium feels all right

Donna enjoys the feeling that comes with competing. If she didn't, she wouldn't have played netball for 25 years. The rather delightful thing about dragon boating is that it's come with a few unexpected rewards. Basically, she's found herself bagging some National Championship medals – paddling in crews that have done well enough to achieve a podium finish, and more than once, if you don't mind! At the 2022 National Championships, she and her crew mates came away with three silver medals – one in the women's, one in the mixed, and one in the team pursuit. Yes, that's right, the team pursuit. Two crews per team – a men's and a women's – combining forces to compete a course faster than the opposition.

If you're reading this and thinking that dragon boating medals aren't significant, think again. Dragon boat crews take their sport seriously. In Donna's case, the National Championship training program included twice-weekly training sessions and several trips to train on the magnificent Manning River, in Taree. There's dedication in these boats, and whilst the crews might be of an older age bracket, there's no lack of desire. Dragon boating is a true team sport. In fact, it's a capital 'T' team sport. After all, how many sports have up to 22 team members contributing at the same time? Not many we can think of. This is an element of dragon boating Donna greatly enjoys.

The here and now

Another aspect she loves about dragon boating is the way it pulls her into the here and now. The way it requires her to concentrate, to stay focused on keeping the rhythm of the boat. In netball, if you lose your concentration, you risk a ball to the back of the head. In dragon boating, there's a chance you'll get hit with a paddle and so it pays to keep your 'head in the boat'. For Donna, the great thing about this is you get a chance to (temporarily) forget about every worry and hassle in your life. You get to park them at the pontoon and paddle the boat out, where the only concern is synchronising with your crew mates and building boat speed.

As a result, by the time she returns from a paddle, Donna's mind is clear and she generally has a fresh perspective on anything that might have been concerning her. This makes paddling an important way of keeping her grounded and balanced. It has taught her how to be disciplined, patient, and still – all things that contribute positively to other aspects of her life.

The social side of the sport

As we chatted to Donna about her love of dragon boating, one thing kept coming up: the social side of the sport. As much as Donna enjoys the feeling of competition, she really values the connection with others and the experience of working as a team. And this is something that appears to be rather distinctive about dragon boating. As she explained, whilst the sport does attract younger (under 40 years old) paddlers, the majority are older, people looking to keep moving, do it in interesting ways, and perhaps expand their social networks. Parents who are empty nesters, residents new to an area, or sporty-types looking for a new challenge (as Donna was). Dragon boating attracts them all, and that's something she really loves.

You see, Donna is a connector. She's a social facilitator at heart, someone who has the energy to create situations that people benefit from. This was one of the reasons she decided to run for club President. She likes to make things social, likes thinking about onshore activities that can make dragon boating much more than a sport. A sport that can create a sense of belonging. The feeling that people are part of something, and have something motivating them to get up and out in the morning. Whilst netball provided a great social vibe, she's found it's a stronger vibe with dragon boaters. Why? Demographics mostly. Her netballer friends tended to be younger, with busier lives. Her dragon boat friends have a little more time and a little more inclination – or opportunity – to be social. So, there's a great feeling that surrounds their club.

The inspiration side of the sport

There's a perception that dragon boating is a sport dominated by women who've survived breast cancer. It's true that the sport is especially popular amongst women. When we asked her about it,

Donna estimated a split of 70% women and 30% men, although the sport is gender diverse. But it attracted participation from women who are living with, or have lived through, a breast cancer experience. Without having talked about that at length, the allure of dragon boating to these women makes sense: A large team of people striving towards a shared goal. A positive, supportive social group, and a sense of belonging. After the perils of what can be a terminal diagnosis, it's hard to imagine a more enriching environment.

Extreme Ironing

What is it?

Extreme ironing is an adventure sport that involves attempting to successfully undertake a common domestic task – ironing – in locations that are either remote, relatively inaccessible, or in some other way practically challenging. This has seen enthusiasts undertake ironing in locations as diverse as forests, alpine areas, and even underwater, or whilst standing on car rooves or ice sheets, or when skydiving or water skiing.

Now, it is not our aim to convince you that extreme ironing is widely practiced. It isn't. Of all the physical pursuits in this book, it is arguably the most unusual. We are merely alerting you to its existence and want to point out three things that distinguish extreme ironing from other sports and physical pursuits. First, the sport thrives on the *imagination* of its participants. Ironing was successfully undertaken on water skis because someone imagined it could be done. Second, their imagination was matched by *creativity*. Having seen the possibility, they worked out how to organise the use of an iron and ironing board aboard the back of a speedboat. Finally, they put together a *plan* and had the audacity to execute it.

Imagination, creativity, planning: the qualities you need if you want to iron whilst water skiing, or hang gliding, or cycling. It's a sport where the logistical challenges are a constant, and might explain its appeal to an increasing number of people.

What are its origins?

Extreme ironing appears to have originated in the UK somewhere between 1980 and 1997. Some credit Tony Hiam with having created the sport in 1980, in Yorkshire, whilst others award Phil Shaw (a.k.a. 'Steam'), from Leicester, that honour. Despite its debatable origins, by 2002 this form of ironing had become so popular, it was given its own World Championship event. A total of 12 teams took part in the first event, with competitors having the option to compete in five different sections: urban, water, forest, lauda (climbing-wall), and freestyle.

Soon after, in 2003, the profile of this unusual physical pursuit was raised, following the release of Phil Shaw's book *Extreme Ironing*. This landmark publication gave readers a general introduction to the sport, with examples of various feats of ironing that had been accomplished up to that time. Since then, it has seen an increase in popularity, and with it the creation of many world records. These include an elevation record set by a British group that ironed a Union Jack above Mt Everest basecamp (5,440 metres), and a depth record set by an Italian free diver who ironed a t-shirt in the world's deepest pool (42 metres). A variety of team ironing records also exist, such as the 2011 underwater record set by a group of 173 divers in the Netherlands.

What rules, if any, does it have?

To qualify for a world record in extreme ironing, the following rules apply:
- Ironing boards must conform to a standard size of one metre in length and 30 cm in width.
- The board must have legs.
- The irons must be made of traditional materials, with an iron base (not the more modern hard-plastic models).
- Garments of any type and size can be ironed, provided they are not smaller than a tea towel.

The joy of it all

Aimee is a 38-year-old office administrator. She works in the real estate industry, the world of private homes and commercial properties. Aimee quite enjoys real estate, but it's nothing compared to the enjoyment she gets from the world outside those homes and properties. She adores being outdoors. In particular, she loves the landscape of the Blue Mountains, a region of the Great Diving Range located 50 km west of Sydney.

One of the reasons Aimee loves this area is that it's the canyon capital of Australia. In her mind, there's nowhere better to go canyoning, which is something that she, and her friends, do whenever they can. In many ways, Aimee organises her life around canyoning. She competes courses on it, reads as much as she can about it, plans trips, posts regularly on social media, and– she's even become a qualified guide, so she can share this joy with others.

So, if Aimee is into canyoning so much, why is she featured in a chapter on extreme ironing? That's easy. Plenty of extreme ironing has happened in canyons, and Aimee has pressed her fair share of t-shirts and tea towels to make her reflections an excellent addition to the book. Plus, as far as passion for her sport goes, there are few who match her.

A sometimes activity

To be clear, like bog snorkelling, extreme ironing isn't an every-day or even every-week activity. As it happens, Aimee has only performed extreme ironing about seven or eight times. But she and her friends have enjoyed the uniqueness of it, along with all the imagination, creativity, and planning it entails. Truth be told, it's more usual for them to go canyoning in fancy dress costumes – to rock climb up or abseil down waterfalls, slide through crevices, and plunge into rivers dressed as princesses, Halloween characters, the Tiger King, or one of Santa's elves. They enjoy this extra dimension of their sport and, currently, they are kicking around an idea of extreme ironing whilst canyoning, and doing it in extremely high heels.

Whilst extreme ironing is an occasional activity for Aimee, canyoning is not. She canyons every weekend, pretty much without fail. On the rare occasions when she can't (as happened a couple of times during COVID-19 lockdowns), she gets quite restless. Canyoning plays a vital role in her life and has an almost addictive quality. But it wasn't always like this. Ten years ago, Aimee was, by her own admission, 'a bit of a princess', and had zero interest in doing the things she does now.

An urban existence

Aimee grew up in the western suburbs of Sydney. She was never an especially sporty kid and, aside from her parents' interest in plants, she didn't have much experience with nature settings. By the time she was working, Aimee lived a decidedly urban existence, working mainly to finance her social life, partying a good deal, and had a regular gym habit. She measured her success by how well she felt she was doing, compared to others.

All of this amounted to a not very satisfying life and she had really struggled to find 'her place'. For Aimee, genuine and fulfilling friendships had been very hard to find. As a result, she was left not really knowing what was missing, and only knowing that things weren't quite right. As a result, her mental health suffered, and she battled with depression.

Things changed a bit once she reached her thirties and began to do a bit of bushwalking. For the first time in her life, she felt a connection to the natural world. As far as she can recall, this wasn't triggered by anything specific; she just got curious about hiking and started exploring it. She bought some books, did some reading, and got out and walked as much as she could. Aimee found she quite liked it, as it gave her some respite from the demands of city living.

Finding your tribe and making it count

Personal change happens at different speeds. Sometimes fast, sometimes slow. When a period of rapid change occurs, its usually on the back of a longer, much slower period of change – a time when your dissatisfaction, sadness, annoyance, frustration, and/ or lack of purpose can grow to such an extent that when the right opportunity comes your way, you grab it with both hands. That's what happened for Aimee. After a decade of dissatisfaction, she knew she wasn't living her best life. Not even close. Most disconcertingly, she felt she had yet to find her people and was keen to do so.

This all changed in 2019, when she signed up to do a group canyoning tour. Although she signed up willingly, she didn't think she was going to like it. The idea of getting her hair wet and being cold did not appeal to her. But, how wrong she was, as it turned out. She did the tour and loved every minute of it. It was instantaneous. Somehow, she'd stumbled on something she desperately needed, but had never been able to identify.

Whilst there are lots of things she loves about canyoning, one of the best is that it helped her to find 'her people'. A tribe that she could really connect with. And having done that, Aimee was out to make up for lost time.

Recreational misfits?

Aimee threw herself into canyoning with vigour. Unlike Sydney, where good friendships had proved difficult to come by, Aimee found the canyoning community easy. She immediately felt at home amongst people who were adventurous, warm, and outgoing, and had a healthy dose of crazy. A good kind of crazy. The sort that people have when they they're looking to 'suck the marrow out of life'. People for whom more conventional physical pursuits aren't quite satisfying enough. Recreational misfits, if you like.

The canyoning community embraced Aimee in a way she had never experienced before. Although she completed some basic skills courses, most of her learning was self-directed and supported by the people she did trips with. This meant she had some great mentors, people who really helped her get the most out of the sport. This allowed her to get in and out of some awe-inspiring country, country that most people never get to see: Pristine mountain forests with stunning waterfalls and crystal-clear water. Places that deliver an adrenaline rush getting in to, because of the risk, followed by an intense sense of satisfaction and contentment when you're there, because of the beauty. Places that also deliver that special kind of cold-water therapy only waterfalls can provide, and invigorate every fibre in your body.

Yes, Aimee loves canyoning. For her, it's now an essential part of life. It provides her with a constant source of physical challenge and scaffolds her mental health. Canyon country is like a spiritual home. Exploring it balances her and provides places she can escape to with other recreational misfits and, if the washing basket is full, even get some ironing done…

Fencing

What is it?

Fencing is a semi-contact duelling sport, as it involves two opponents facing off, with weapons, and engaging in combat according to an accepted procedure. In fencing, the weapon is a sword, or, more accurately, three swords: a foil, a sabre, and an epee. The aim of all three fencing disciplines is the same: to score more points than an opponent through strikes or 'hits' to the body. But each weapon has a different construction and weight. Each also has a different use strategy, as the target zone for the foil is the torso, the sabre targets the torso and arms, and the epee is permitted to target the whole body. Although some recreational fencers compete in all three disciplines, most elite-level fencers specialise in only one of the three.

Fencing is highly technical and intense. It requires a sharp mind and a limber body, so much so that it has been compared to simultaneously playing chess and running a 100-metre sprint. Mentally, it's a battle of wits, with opponents trying to outthink each other and implement strategies designed to reveal defensive weaknesses and offensive opportunities. Physically, it's a type of dance, with the combatants trying to remain light and well balanced, such that they can quickly coordinate their hands, feet, and torso during offensive and defensive movements.

What are its origins?

The use of swords dates back to the Bronze Age (ca. 1600 BC) and their emergence as an evolution of the dagger. Used for a variety of purposes, including hunting, swords are nonetheless best known as a weapon of war and were used as recently as World War I. However, with the evolution of firearms, military sword use has steadily diminished over the past two hundred years and they now have mostly ceremonial and symbolic significance. Despite this, a broader interest in swordplay and sword fighting led to the development of competitive (non-fatal) forms of sport and recreation. This occurred in the mid-18th century with the emergence of several fencing academies and schools across Europe. Whilst initially a fashionable sport for the aristocracy, the codification of its basic techniques and rules during the 19th century saw it become more widespread and it was included in 1896 as a sport in the first Summer Olympic Games of the modern era. This makes fencing one of the oldest Olympic sports, and one of only five events to have been included in every modern Games thus far.

What rules, if any, does it have?

Fencing's rules relate to scoring, safety, and etiquette. The scoring rules are specific to the discipline involved, with points in the foil, sabre, and epee scored based on how many hits are landed in the target zones of each discipline. Points can also only be scored within the marked boundaries of the piste (playing area), which is 14 metres long and 1.5–2.0 metres wide. The safety rules are extremely important, as fencing is a semi-contact sport that involves offensively thrusting a weapon. As such, some standard protective equipment is required to avoid injury, including a helmet that fully covers the head, with a tough mesh mask to protect the eyes, a protective jacket and pants, and a glove worn on the weapon hand. The etiquette rules include the saluting of an opponent and the referee before and after a bout, no physical contact or barging, and no use of the non-sword arm or hand to cover target zones.

The joy of it all

Eddie is a 58-year-old casual academic, the owner of a fencing business, and a Level 1 fencing coach. Whilst he is very knowledgeable about the sport, he'd only been fencing for just over nine years when we spoke. You could say that Eddie genuinely was a late starter. But he's developed such a passion for the sport that it's become an important part of his life.

Life as a 'fencing dad'

Eddie's interest in sport is a relatively recent development. In fact, for the first 50 of his 58 years, it didn't feature at all. He grew up in a family with little interest in sport and who provided little encouragement to seek it out. In addition, Eddie was skinnier and lighter than most kids his age, which made school sports a bit of a struggle, and made him the target of some bullying. As a result, he devoted much of his adolescence and free time to music, which continued into early adulthood. As a result, he is a multi-instrumentalist who plays the piano, viola, trombone, and mandolin.

Eddie's distance from sport may well have continued, were it not for his sons. Around the time they became teenagers, there was a need to find them a physical pursuit they could channel their energy into and give them a focus. After his younger son announced he wanted to do 'sword-fighting', Eddie contacted the local fencing club and made an enquiry. He was quite happy to do this because his niece had taken up the sport a few years earlier, and so he knew a little about it. He started taking his youngest son to weekly fencing classes. Although the boy didn't stick with it for long, his older brother did, and Eddie became a fencing dad.

He'd go along and watch, without getting involved. That is, until one night, after about a year, when he decided to give it a try.

You just never know!

To his surprise, Eddie enjoyed it immediately. There were a few reasons for this. First, a fencing foil is surprisingly light (only 500 grams). As soon as he picked it up, he felt capable of using it, because it didn't require a lot of upper body or arm strength. Second, very quickly after starting to fence, he found himself landing hits. This increased his confidence, because he felt he'd found a sport he could do. Plus, having watched his son at fencing club for about a year, he was already familiar with how it was done.

In addition, fencing provided him with a solid aerobic workout. Although Eddie had never been much for organised sport, he had tried various things over the years to create a base of fitness for himself. He'd played some tennis, bought an exercise bike once, and done a little running – yet none of it for long periods of time. Fencing was different. Not only did it suit his lighter, slighter body type, it was also a great aerobic workout. The bouts are short, but very intense. (If you need any evidence of this, just search up an Olympic fencing bout.) Eddie is now fitter than he's ever been.

The DIY training program

Eddie knew that a key to enjoying his new sport was to make sure that he was fit enough. He paid close attention to how other people trained, observed the warmup routines of other fencers before bouts, got ideas from people in chat rooms and fencing workshops, watched videos about strength training, and even got some inspiration from the local soccer team. Over the course of several years, Eddie developed a training program for himself that includes an array of dynamics stretches, body strengthening exercises, and mobility drills such as star jumps, lunges, high knees, butt kicks, lateral lunges, and grapevines. His DIY program has become an indispensable part of his sport and his enjoyment of it.

This DIY program highlights something else about Eddie that is critical to his enjoyment of fencing. By his own admission, he's a big-picture thinker. That is, when he decides to do something, he likes to understand what he's doing. Indeed, his first job was as a research assistant and he has a PhD, so he's used to analysis and enjoys it, which is a good thing, because when it comes to fencing, there's a lot you can learn.

The technical side of fencing

In order to develop a decent understanding of fencing, you need to learn a bit about its history. The art and skill of the three disciplines, foil, epee, and sabre, are closely connected to the original uses of those weapons. For example, the epee is a sword that was designed for stabbing, whilst the sabre was a slashing weapon used by mounted cavalry. As such, these two disciplines have two different techniques and styles of combat.

For a research-minded person like Eddie, this aspect of the sport made it even more attractive, so much so that when describing these aspects of the sport in our interview, he spoke fluidly and enthusiastically about the sport's history, the weapons' characteristics, and his personal collection (which fencers impressively call an armoury). There was little doubt that this side of the sport has added considerably to his overall enjoyment.

Some time on the podium

Eddie has been fencing now for nine years. Despite finding the sport manageable to start with, it took a while before he achieved any competitive success. But this is what generally happens with most sports, and so it was for Eddie. In fact, it's a good thing he enjoyed the sport so much, because after he began competing in 2015, it took a long time to record his first win, and his first few open competitions resulted in a series of last places. Then, in 2016, he had his first win, and then another, and another. Although he wasn't winning medals yet, he was no longer coming last either, and that was encouragement enough.

Things really turned around for Eddie when he discovered veteran competitions. These were run for competitors aged 40 and over, a category where the fencing was a little more relaxed but still hard fought. Not long after, in his second year of competing, Eddie broke through and won his first medal, a bronze in a veteran epee tournament, followed closely by a silver in the 2016 NSW Veteran Championships. This marked a memorable time in his life. He was fully engaged in a sport, travelling to competitions. Getting up in the early hours of the morning to be on the piste by 9am in Sydney. Learning how to manage his energy needs and fuel himself well. And it was paying off. Albeit not the most naturally gifted athlete, he can more than hold his own. As a result, his win/loss ratio has greatly improved and his medal collection has grown steadily.

A key motivator

It is clear that fencing is a key part of Eddie's life. He sees it as an important source of motivation. It adds an extra dimension to his life and gives him a compelling reason to stay fit. Training not only helps him to keep competing, but it also greatly increases his enjoyment of that. Fencing has also helped him to become more socially engaged. Eddie knows that by virtue of his work and personality, his social world could easily shrink. However, his involvement in fencing propels him into the world – as a competitor, as a coach, and as an administrator and organiser of local events. As such, his social network has expanded greatly, and he has formed some good friendships and made many acquaintances.

For all these reasons, Eddie hopes to continue fencing for some time to come – at least as long as his body permits it. All this from investigating a sport that was never intended for him. What started out as a potential interest for his sons turned into his own interesting and absorbing physical pursuit. It's a sport that opened up a new world for him, and has helped make him a fitter, more knowledgeable, and more socially connected person. That's a lot to gain from any sport.

Goalball

What is it?

Goalball is a fast, dynamic Paralympic sport played by visually impaired athletes. It's an indoor game played on a court roughly the size of a basketball court and combines the ball-rolling skills used in ten-pin bowling with the goalkeeping skills used in soccer. Like soccer, the aim is to score more goals than the opposing team by rolling a 1.25-kg ball, often at speeds of up to 60 km/hr, towards a netted goal on the opposition's baseline. Because the goal spans the entire baseline, the goal is defended by three players.

Although all goalball players must be legally blind to compete, this does not mean they are all completely blind. However, the visual capacity of teams is equalised by having all players wear blackened eye masks. This forces players to track the ball with only their hearing as they try to prevent goal scoring, which they do by listening for the sound of a bell that is located within the ball. This requires the game to be played in silence, without crowd noise, and with players prohibited from communicating when the ball is in motion. To help players position themselves on the court, the floor is marked with lines that are textured and can be felt by the players' hands.

Goalball is unusual as a Paralympic sport, given that it has no mainstream equivalent and was specifically developed as a game for vision-impaired athletes. This is different to wheelchair rugby, which is a direct adaptation of rugby union; or sitting volleyball, which is a direct adaptation of volleyball. Instead, it's a rare example of a sport that caters for the lived realities of its participants and supports greater diversity and inclusion into the world of competitive sport.

What are its origins?

Before goalball was a sport, it was a form of physical rehabilitation. It was created in 1946 by Hanz Lorenzen and Sepp Reindl, as a way to support returning World War II servicemen who had sustained visual injuries in combat. By the 1960s, players were experimenting with different ways to attack and defend, and becoming more skilled with the basics of the game. Over the next few decades, its popularity increased significantly.

Unusually, goalball was recognised at Paralympic level before it had its own World Championships. It was included in 1972 as a demonstration sport at the Heidelberg Paralympic Games. Four years later it debuted as a full Paralympic sport at the 1976 Toronto Games, and two years later, Vocklamarck, Austria, hosted the first World Championships. A significant event in the global organisation of goalball took place in the early 1980s, when the International Blind Sports Association (IBSA) was formed and became the sport's governing body. In the 40 years since, goalball has spread to six continents and, according to the IBSA world rankings, there are currently 97 international men's teams and 60 women's teams.

What rules, if any, does it have?

As mentioned, goalball is a game for people living with visual impairment. The game is fairly straightforward, with a relatively complicated set of rules to keep the game fair and safe. These rules include:
- Wearing opaque eye masks (blindfolds) that are checked when substitutions are made
- Adhering to set playing zones, each three metres deep, that include a team area (for defending), a landing area (for

attacking), and a neutral area, where no play can take place (allowing defenders to hear the ball)
- Remaining silent during periods when the ball is in motion
- Returning the ball into play within 10 seconds of taking possession
- Ensuring the ball contacts the floor before the midline when shooting

When rule violations occur, a team is penalised by requiring the player who committed the offence to defend their goal singlehandedly.

The joy of it all

Tyan is 32-year-old childcare worker. She is also a three-time Australian Paralympic goalball athlete, having represented Australia at the 2012 (London), 2016 (Rio), and 2020 (Tokyo) Paralympic Games. Tyan has recently retired from the sport, and has enjoyed her 12 year career so much that she's now motivated to find ways to give something back to the sport and encourage other athletes to get involved.

Not just making up the numbers

Even though Tyan is legally blind, she is not without a degree of sight. She was born with a condition called ocular albinism, which affects the retina and nerves behind the eyes. Most of what she can see is blurred, so she is unable to detect fine details, and she is sensitive to glare. As you might imagine, this makes many things in life rather challenging, including participating in sport. Despite this, Tyan was highly active as a kid and played mainstream soccer and touch football for many seasons, along with a season of T-ball. Whilst she enjoyed what she did, her vision impairment meant there were some team positions and roles she simply couldn't play. This made the experience of mainstream sport a little frustrating for an enthusiastic kid from a sporty family. Her sight limitations meant she couldn't contribute as much as she'd like, and at times she felt like she was there merely to make up the numbers.

But there was one sport she knew of – goalball – that offered something different. She first came across it at the Sydney 2000 Paralympics. She was keen to give it a try, but at that time it was a new sport and not played anywhere near where she lived. So, she parked the idea and got on with other things.

Then, in 2009, Tyan's vision support teacher was helping her find employment as a disability support worker. During a coffee chat with a potential employer, Tyan was asked if she'd ever played goalball. 'No I haven't', she replied, 'but I'd like to try'. As luck would have it, there was a goalball schools tournament happening soon after and Tyan was encouraged to enter. She acquainted herself with the rules, got a couple of friends together, and joined a team. To their surprise, they won the competition. Although she didn't realise it at the time, this would mark the start of an international career, a career in a sport where her participation was made possible by her vision impairment, not limited by it.

Non-stop burpees

Goalball is a demanding sport. It's fast, highly dynamic, and takes considerable concentration. It also requires a good deal of fitness. As Tyan described it, goalball is like 'doing non-stop burpees'. That's because to score goals, players need to stop the ball, quickly jump to their feet, and after taking a few strides, roll it forcefully towards the opponent's goal. Once a shot on goal has been completed, the player quickly gets ready to defend. They do this by lying on the floor and extending their arms and legs – like a soccer goalkeeper – into a defensive posture that can stop opposition shots by using hands or body blocks.

These are the basic plays in goalball, and they happen many, many times across two 12-minute halves. That's 24 minutes of burpees! A lot of explosive body movement which requires endurance, not something you get without training. We mention this because the physical demands of goalball should not be underestimated. Indeed, the physical challenge is one of the things Tyan loves about the sport.

But that challenge is more than just physical. Imagine this – you're playing a ball sport without the use of your eyes, where your ability to do well depends on you tuning into the sound of a bell inside a ball rocketing towards you. You must be fully switched on and totally in the moment. If you're not – if you're 'off in your head', thinking about other things – you may miss the sound you need to locate a ball that's heading your way.

A synchronisation in play and perspectives

When Tyan first started describing goalball, she talked about it being an integrated sport, with elements of ten-pin bowling, dodgeball, soccer, and synchronised swimming. Pardon? Synchronised swimming? This didn't make a lot of sense to start with, but that soon changed.

Success in goalball relies on good coordination between all six team members, and their ability to synchronise as they substitute in and out of the three-person on-court team. The challenge to coordinate a team of blindfolded players is hardly straightforward. It simply can't be done unless the teammates have a good understanding of each other, high levels of trust, and maintain clear communication (when permitted during a game). When all this happens, the result, according to Tyan, is something akin to synchronised swimming. Who knew?

Tyan has always enjoyed this aspect of the game. Not only has she enjoyed the synchronisation just described, but she really values the lasting relationships the game has provided her – relationships that have improved her knowledge of both the game and her performance. She's also learnt a lot from her teammates, things that've helped her tackle the challenges of life. Whilst the social side of the game is something she will miss, her plan to make non-playing contributions to the game, such as mentoring young players, will keep her connected to people who really matter to her.

Taking disability out of the picture

Clearly, goalball has meant a lot to Tyan. She's loved the physical challenge of it, and the requirement to train as hard as any athlete in a mainstream sport. She's loved being able to get out and experience the world, which competing at the international level has given her. She's also loved forming and maintaining some great friendships, which team sport tends to bring.

Perhaps more than anything else, she loves that goalball took her disability out of the equation. When she started playing at the age of 19, all her sporting experience had been in mainstream sport, trying her best to fit in, despite her visual challenge, and find a way to play. With goalball, that all went away. She could just be Tyan. She wasn't the girl with the weird eyes anymore. She wasn't the girl who had to prove herself to get a spot on the team, and constantly wonder if she was being picked solely because others felt sorry for her. All that doubt was erased.

With goalball, Tyan got picked because she was good at goalball. And, as it turned out, she became one of the best in the country. Not only had she found her sporting 'thing', but Tyan went and made the most of it. And having made the most of it, she's happy now to move on to other things, to get on with life and to throw herself at it, like she would a set of burpees. And who doesn't love a set of burpees?

Hiking

What is it?

In this chapter, hiking is used as a generic term to describe walking for pleasure in a variety of different nature settings and wilderness areas. Such areas can include high mountain country, sub-tropical rainforests, arid scrubland or semi-desert, beaches and coastal wetlands, and river valleys. When people walk in such terrain, they may do so for periods ranging between one and four hours, to longer day walks (five to 10 hours), or multi-day walks that could cover distances of more than 30 kilometres and require overnight camping in tents or huts.

We should clarify that hiking is the term used in the United States and Canada for recreational walking. Other countries use other terms. For example, British walkers are more likely to call it fell-walking, whilst Australians go bushwalking, and New Zealanders go tramping. They all mean roughly the same thing and reflect the preoccupation that human beings have with nature, and our keenness to spend time in it.

What are its origins?

Walking is the most natural and basic form of human transportation. For millennia, we have relied on foot power to hunt, forage, explore new territories, and otherwise move about over land. Indeed, walking for prolonged periods has always had a clear purpose, like securing food, religious pilgrimages, exploring new lands, or traditional rites of passage (such as the physical and spiritual 'walkabout' journeys used for thousands of years by the First Nations people of Australia).

The idea of walking for pleasure has a much shorter history. Evidence of recreational walking can be traced back to the 11th century, but it wasn't until the late 18th century that it became popular in Europe and North America. This was the time of the Industrial Revolution, when heavy industry, machine manufacturing, and rapid urbanisation was transforming the western world. It was also the time of the Romantic era, when literary figures like Wordsworth, Keats, Emerson, and Thoreau reacted to these changes by noting the beauty in nature, and publishing essays inspired by their walking tours.

Towards the end of the 19th century, walking clubs emerged, gaining popularity amongst those keen to escape the cramped, unsanitary conditions of large cities. This was further supported in the UK by 'right to roam' legislation that legalised access to certain privately owned land, lakes, and rivers, and in the US through the creation of an extensive network of national parks and protected wilderness areas.

What rules, if any, does it have?

Hiking is not considered a competitive sport. As such, there are no rules to summarise. Rather, there appears to be some universally accepted 'trail etiquette' that applies to all forms of walking in nature, regardless of duration. This includes:

- Keeping noise to a minimum, by speaking quietly and managing technology
- Giving way to uphill traffic, as going up is generally harder than going down
- Cleaning up after yourself and leaving no trace of your visit
- Walking on designated trails and not damaging natural habitat by 'bush crashing'
- Being friendly and helpful to other walkers

- Maximising personal safety by walking with at least one other person, carrying a locator beacon, planning well, and choosing walks that are matched to one's level of fitness.

The joy of it all

Eleanor is a 63-year-old registered nurse. She grew up in New Zealand and has fond memories of being surrounded by beautiful countryside. She also remembers walking with her father, who was a keen hiker and an even keener observer of the natural world. As such, Eleanor learned that hiking was about more than just getting from point A to point B. It was an exercise in noticing nature and being curious about it. Although she never got to do any of the big, multi-day walks her father went on, these early experiences established nature in Eleanor's mind as a happy and positive place.

Tramping, if you don't mind!

Now, being a New Zealander, Eleanor refers to her much-loved physical pursuit as tramping.

But when she was 11 years old, her family moved to Australia. This meant she became a bushwalker, which meant a change in terrain but no change in enjoyment. She found the Australian flora and fauna intriguing and, as she did in New Zealand, whenever she ventured into the Australian bush, it was to complete shorter, same-day walks.

This was the way she did it for over 30 years. Whilst the bushwalking wasn't always as regular a pastime as Eleanor would have liked, whenever she could get outdoors in this way, she always found it thoroughly rewarding. But there was one thing she hadn't ever tried – a multi-day walk, a walk where you 'have to carry everything on your back, like a turtle', as she described it, including clothes, food, water, cooking equipment, and if walking a track with no huts, a tent. This was a personal aspiration that'd been forming for years, but the timing had just never been right. Ironically, when the time was right, New Zealand was where it happened.

The adventure that just kept on giving

In 2005, at the age of 47, Eleanor decided to attempt her first multi-day hike, a decision that was made quickly. All it took was a short conversation with her aunt and uncle, who had just booked a trip to go walking in New Zealand. When they suggested Eleanor join them, it 'flipped a switch' inside of her. Before she knew it, she'd booked a ticket, purchased some gear, and was on a plane heading for New Zealand to walk the 63-km Rees and Dart Track.

For Eleanor this trip had both elements needed to qualify as an adventure: It had perceived risk (could she do it?), and an uncertain outcome (how would it go?). Whilst a little nervous, she was reassured by the confidence of her companions. Her aunt and uncle had done their research, seemed well organised, and although 20 years her senior, were energetic and enthusiastic. Unfortunately, once on the trail, this wasn't enough. By the end of the first day, her uncle had struggled so badly he had to be airlifted out the next morning. This left Eleanor in the middle of nowhere, minus her walking partners, with only two options: (i) retrace her steps and walk back out, or (ii) push on and keep moving forward.

In many ways this was the worst imaginable outcome. She was naturally concerned about her uncle, and this strange reality had pushed her even further outside her comfort zone. Fortunately, the track was quite busy that week and she quickly met a very encouraging, confident Australian couple who offered to join her for day two. That was hugely helpful, but it didn't change the physical demands of carrying a pack for hours over challenging terrain, or the mental challenges that came with that.

The personal triumph of Cascade Saddle

Now, as often happens, adversity can lead to triumph. This arrived on the third day. Sticking to her original plan, Eleanor decided to do the out-and-back day walk to an area of renowned beauty. The problem was that she would have to do it alone, as her day two companions had a different plan. Not that this stopped her. She'd already been quite bold, and it was time to be bolder.

The next morning, Eleanor got up very early and left the hut at first light. She felt this was important to do, as being a slow walker, she was concerned she'd be outpaced by others and wind up being the last person on the track at the end of the day. As predicted, it was a challenging day, with 10 hours of walking and lots of firsts, like scrambling over large boulders and rocky stream crossings, and trying to get back to the hut before nightfall. Her walk to Cascade Saddle and back was arduous and exhausting, but, as she insists, so worthwhile. The views were awe inspiring, the satisfaction immense. More than anything else, it was a reward she had wholly earned – earned through persistence, self-reliance, and her own foot power! That day, more than any other, was the day she understood just how wonderful hiking could be. It's a day she still counts as one of the most memorable of her life.

The value of grit and determination

For Eleanor, hiking is a special way to see the world. She likes that by relying solely on her feet, she can get to places and see things that wouldn't be possible any other way. Experiences she has to earn the right to enjoy, by putting in some effort and working hard. In this way, walking is a good metaphor for life, so hiking carries a deeper meaning for Eleanor. She likes the physical challenge that it brings and relishes the chance to test herself. Ever since that first multi-day walk in New Zealand, this attitude, she says, has been 'snowballing'.

Whilst Eleanor really enjoys long walks in nature, she doesn't feel she has obvious talent for it or clear physical gifts. What she does have is lots of 'sheer, bloody-minded determination' and grit. She has a strong drive to visit as many special places in the world as her feet can manage. Not especially agile or particularly fast, she is, however, good at planning her walks and is always very committed to completing them. And going slowly is not a disadvantage. It means she gets to notice more, just like she did as a young girl. It also makes walking an exercise in mindfulness, an activity that involves heightened awareness of, and attention to, the natural world. An activity that's good for her body, mind, and spirit. An activity that helps her remember that she's but a small part of a much bigger universe, which she finds a comforting thought. It comes with a sense of gratitude and good fortune, and a continuing desire to keeping on hiking (pardon, *tramping*) for as long as she can. Indeed, if she could pick the manner of her passing, she'd like it to be when she's 95, lying face down on a track with a pack on her back – just like a turtle.

Oh, the people you meet!

In the 15-plus years she's been a committed multi-day walker, Eleanor and her partner, Denis, have hiked in Australia and New Zealand. Everywhere they've gone, they have met incredible people, often when staying overnight in track huts. People who are warm and friendly and come from interesting and diverse backgrounds. People who value the environment and appreciate its many gifts. People who are unerringly helpful and willing to assist when assistance is needed – just like day two on the Rees and Dart Track.

She's also been inspired by what many of these people can do, especially some of the older walkers. Although hard to determine how much hiking might contribute to their overall strength, agility, balance, and speed, she reckons it must be a fair bit. As such, these people are a powerful reminder of the critical role that physical activity plays in healthy ageing. Given the joy and satisfaction that Eleanor gets from hiking, these people are also important role models. After all, if there's to be any hope of her gloriously departing this earth at the age of 95, lying face down on a track, she'll need to be able to get out onto the track. As unconventional as that goal might be, if it helps produce more Cascade Saddle experiences, then why not?

Ice Skating

What is it?

Ice skating is a form of self-propulsion that involves gliding across an icy surface with bladed skates. This makes it a highly challenging activity, as the movements are performed on a smooth, low-friction surface with a reduced base of support (as blades are narrower than feet). This makes ice skating – like skiing – rather an unnatural thing to do and quite challenging to learn. However, given it is such an unusual way to move through space, ice skating is a popular form of recreation. It is also the basis of at least three different competitive sports: figure skating, speed skating (short and long track), and ice hockey.

Figure skating is very technical and aesthetically pleasing. It involves the execution of a sequence of highly technical movements, performed in time to music. In this way it resembles dancing and gymnastics, and like both, is judged according to how precisely a skater executes set movements. In contrast, speed skating focuses primarily on velocity and the time taken to travel a set distance in one direction. As with track running in athletics, skaters can compete over a variety of short sprint distances which are powerful and explosive, or longer distances that rely on movement efficiency and speed endurance. In the team sport of ice hockey, the skating is fast and furious, and used to create offensive and defensive plays that can assist a team to score more goals than their opposition.

What are its origins?

Ice skating has existed for thousands of years, with evidence suggesting it may have first been used as a form of transportation in southern Finland. This makes good sense. Ice has a low coefficient of friction, which means less force is needed to create and maintain motion. As such, skating is more energy efficient than walking or running, and covers distance a good deal faster. Unsurprisingly, the practice of skating on ice became widespread across many of the colder regions of the world, initially on blades made of bone, and then of wood. A significant turning point came around the 16th century, when some skates were made with blades of sharpened steel. This fundamentally changed how people skated, with each stride changing from a glide *on the ice* to a cut *into the ice*, which enabled more power to be generated. This change also led to a steady increase in its popularity, from a pastime initially reserved for members of the upper class to a physical pursuit that could be enjoyed by all, regardless of social standing.

What rules, if any, does it have?

Unlike competitive speed skating, where success is measured in minutes and seconds, competitive figure skating aims to score more points than other skaters. This occurs through the subjective assessment of expert judges. However, to manage that subjectivity, panels of up to 9 judges are used, with consensus scoring determined by removing the lowest and highest scores given for each routine performed. Scoring is based on factors such as grace, flair, control, and musical interpretation. Some basic rules include:

- An expectation that skaters will perform a specific set of movements (such as jumps and turns) a specific number of times

- The use of musical selections that are deemed appropriate for the sport
- The use of costumes that are not excessively decorated or too physically revealing
- The completion of routines within a specific period of time (about two minutes)

The joy of it all

Aylin is a 56-year-old organisational psychologist. Her first experience of ice skating came when she was 13 and had to pick a school sport. Liking the look of it, Aylin though she'd give it a go, and can still vividly recall lacing up a pair of skates for the first time. Then she stepped onto the ice – and took to it immediately. Whilst most people tend to falter, slip, and stumble at first, that wasn't Aylin's experience. She was able to get around the rink with relative ease, helped no doubt by the fact that she knew how to roller skate. But she found that being on the ice was different, and so much better – it felt smoother and more fluid Right from that first day, she adored the sport.

Not long afterwards, Aylin purchased her first pair of skates. They were second-hand and a little too small, but good enough to get started with. And because she was a motivated self-starter, Aylin told her parents she was going to get some coaching. Keen to make skating more than just a school sport, she contacted a coach and arranged her first lesson. But the lesson didn't happen, because there was a mix-up and they never found each other. Disappointed but undeterred, she tried again. Discouragingly, the second meeting never happened either. Why? She's not sure. Maybe the coach didn't think she was serious? Maybe she should have tried harder to find him by asking the skaters who were on the ice? She'll never know.

As she stood waiting at the rink that day – watching skaters, parents, and coaches come and go – she felt a little daunted. Although she really wanted to be involved in this beautiful, glamourous sport, it seemed a little hard to break into. Everyone seemed to know everyone else, and with no background in ice skating, she felt very much like an outsider, and this resulted in her pulling back from pursuing formal lessons. However, she did keep skating at school and for fun, until she was about 19 years old. After that, she stopped, as life went and 'got all busy' on her.

Should auld acquaintance be forgot

Twenty years would pass before Aylin found her way back to a skating rink. During that time, she had completed a university degree, become a psychologist, got married, began a career, and started a family. But being busy didn't mean she'd been inactive – far from it. A perennially active person, Aylin had spent those years running, playing soccer, going to the gym, and doing lots of walking.

Then, just as 2009 was about to transition into 2010, she found herself at a New Year's Eve party, talking to a friend. And, as people do on NYE, they were chatting about their lives: what they'd been doing, and what they planned to do. Amid all that, the topic of sport was raised and, 'like a bolt out of the blue', she found herself talking about ice skating again. This time not as a teenager but as a 42-year-old who'd not been on skates for 20 years. It was a conversation that really got her thinking. Not being someone afflicted by self-directed ageism, when Aylin flirted with the idea of maybe taking it up again, she thought: *Why not?* Why not, indeed. Much like her 13-year-old self, she turned her interest into a plan.

Getting her skates on

Having resolved to start skating again, Aylin took immediate action. One of the first things she did was rent a pair of skates and get some time on the ice. As she had maintained an active lifestyle and kept herself reasonably fit, this wasn't as physically demanding as it might otherwise have been. Importantly, she realised her enjoyment of skating was still intact. So, she bought a pair of skates and went looking for a coach – again. Happily, the third-time-lucky rule applied. She found a coach and, as they say, the rest is history!

There are several things about skating that Aylin particularly enjoys. First, it requires every type of athletic ability. To skate well, she has had to develop strength, flexibility, core stability, cardio endurance, joint mobility, coordination, and balance. As such, skating gives her a full-body workout like nothing else she's ever done. Second, she finds skating endlessly interesting and continually varied. Interesting and varied because of its performance elements, which Aylin has some background in, through musical theatre. Having tread the boards with the local musical society, she's accustomed to dressing up and performing to music. The third thing is the music itself. Aylin loves working with her coach on choosing a piece of music and shaping a routine around it and then, when the pressure is on, executing it on the ice.

That's quite a lot to enjoy – the athletic challenge, the performance, the costumes, the music. For Aylin, ice skating brings several interests together into one complete package.

Oberstdorf!

After starting with her coach, Aylin threw herself into her new sport. She has never found getting around a rink especially difficult, but there's a big difference between doing it for fun and doing it competitively. And because Aylin wanted to compete, this meant nothing less than learning how to dance on ice. So, she got busy with her coach and started focusing on bringing her skating up to a competitive level. They worked on her technique and, bit by bit, developed a routine they felt was good enough to be evaluated by a panel of judges. Eight months after starting, Aylin made her competitive debut in a small, local competition.

Although she doesn't clearly remember how she went, it must not have been too bad, because 10 months later, she was at it again, this time at her first international event, in faraway Oberstdorf, Germany. This gave her something else to love about ice skating – the opportunity to travel.

The psychology of skating

Being a psychologist, the mental side of skating is a constant source of fascination for Aylin. All aspects of performing are of interest to her. There are the pre-performance challenges of building her self-confidence and managing strong emotions, the performance challenges of maintaining full focus, remaining in the moment, and dealing with pressure that is intensified by the requirement to perform solo. But there are also the post-performance challenges of having to constantly take on feedback and being humble enough to accept it and learn from it.

But this is something Aylin has learnt to value. Indeed, skating seems to benefit her work in some important ways. For one, she rarely experiences panic. When faced with a difficult situation, she often reflects on her skating and remembers that 'nothing is as difficult as skating, or as hard as a skating program'. She finds this a comforting thought. It helps to ground her and focus her mind, then muster the determination needed to deal with whatever she's faced with. It was also a crucial counterbalance whilst studying for her doctorate. Earning any PhD is challenging, but doing it part-time whilst also working added to the mental, physical, and emotional challenges. Skating helped her to regularly unhook from those challenges by immersing herself in the delights of skating for a few hours. It was a critical energy management strategy.

Skating is life

The final thing that Aylin enjoys about ice skating is the community it brings her into contact with. She's found them to be an incredibly supportive group of people, genuinely encouraging and invested in the success of anyone who decides to take up the sport. Maybe that's a reflection of two things: the fact that the sport is difficult to master, and that she took it up in her forties. Whatever the reasons, she's found the social side of skating to be hugely enriching, and something she's seen other late starters benefit from.

For all these reasons, Aylin wants skating to be part of her life for as long as she can do it. It provides a connection to her physical self that delivers a whole lot more than simple fitness, not the least of which is the feeling during and after a good performance: a sense of being smooth, fluid, and fast, followed by elation, pride, and intense satisfaction. The joy of working hard and getting a good result. Just as it should be, in life.

Judo

What is it?

Judo is both a martial art and a competitive sport. It is a system of unarmed combat that rose to prominence in late 19th century Japan and has deep historical and philosophical roots. The literal translation of judo is 'gentle way', and reflects the way the art distinguishes itself from other physical disciplines that existed at that time. Most notably, judo removed striking and weapons from close combat, and placed a strong emphasis on free sparring, rather than the disciplined rehearsing of different form movements (i.e., attacking and defensive poses).

The aim in judo is to force an opposing player – a judoka – to yield, by grappling, throwing, wrestling, and pinning that opponent to the floor. A player can win in one of three ways. First, they can score an ippon, which immediately ends the contest. This happens when a full point is awarded after a player throws their opponent onto their back with power *and* control. Alternatively, an ippon can also be awarded if an opponent's shoulders are pinned to the mat for at least 20 seconds. The second way of winning is by scoring two waza-ari (half points) by throwing an opponent with power *or* control, or by maintaining a pin for between 10 and 19 seconds. Finally, in adult matches only, a bout will end if a strangle or armlock results in the submission of one of the players.

What are its origins?

The origins of judo are exclusively linked to one person, Jigoro Kano, who developed the sport towards the end of the 19th century. Kano had an interest in martial arts from an early age, especially jujitsu, a form of close combat used by 17th century Japanese warriors. Unfortunately, jujitsu was becoming unfashionable just at the time Kano wished to pursue it. As such, he had a great deal of trouble finding teachers. But when he did, he studied its art so diligently that, by the age of 22, he was accomplished enough to open his own school and teach. As Kano gained experience as a teacher, he developed his ideas about the art form. He was very interested in the efficiency of human movement, and how, in close combat situations, good technique makes it possible for less physically strong opponents to succeed over stronger ones.

In Kano's view, skilful players should be able to use technique to turn the strength of an opponent against them, causing them to lose balance, power, and control. As the art developed to become a sport, the principle that 'softness controls hardness' was codified in the rules of the sport, as both a means of creating competitive advantage and a pathway for self-development. As it turned out, the physical and philosophical aspects of judo made it broadly appealing and helped it to spread rapidly during the first half of the 20th century. Rather appropriately, it achieved full Olympic status at the 1964 summer games in Tokyo, yet whilst Japan has dominated the overall medal count, judokas from 56 nations on five continents have won Olympics medals. As such, judo can claim to be a truly global sport.

What rules, if any, does it have?

Judo has a complex set of rules and etiquette that determines how points are scored and how players should engage with each other during bouts and more generally conduct themselves. The rules are important for making the sport fair and safe, but etiquette is arguably more important in that it gives judo relevance to good and ethical living. This includes always showing respect for opponents and referees by bowing before and after any contest. It also includes maintaining the spirit of Rei, which reflects the value of always demonstrating self-mastery, ensuring that contests do not descend into violent struggles or fights. Examples of more formal competition rules include:

- No punching or kicking an opponent, or touching their face
- The elbow joint is the only joint that can be the focus of an attack
- Players will be penalised for becoming too defensive, or stalling during bouts
- No negative body gestures or foul language are permitted

The joy of it all

Shane is a 56-year-old schoolteacher and experienced sports administrator. He's been a judoka since he was eight, after he got into a fight at school and came off second best. Sometime later, following the suggestion of a boy who lived nearby, he went to the local dojo and had a try at judo. He liked it immediately. Like most boys, he found that wrestling on a judo mat was great fun. And that's how Shane often describes what judokas do: they wrestle. Strictly speaking he's right, because judo doesn't involve any punching or kicking, just grappling and throwing, which makes it the sporting cousin of wrestling.

After learning the basics of the sport, Shane started to compete at the age of 10. Although not a natural competitor, he developed his sports craft gradually and won a tournament three years later. More success soon followed. He made his first state team by the age of 13, and the national team at 18. This kicked off an 11-year international judo career that saw him compete in tournaments all over the world, including the University World Championship, although not the Olympics.

A great strength and conditioning system

Throughout these years, Shane has had two sporting loves: judo and rugby league. Fortunately, these fitted together well, as judo was helpful for his general strength and conditioning, and also improved his rugby league tackling technique. In fact, judo proved to be ideal training for that. As Shane pointed out, because the sport doesn't involve punching or kicking, a judoka relies on body positioning, weight transfer, and the release of pressure to create competitive advantages on the mat. As such, judokas learn that physical strength is never a decisive advantage.

Rather, they learn that whenever opponents push by using their body weight and strength, two responses are possible. The first and obvious response is to oppose the force by trying to match it, thus creating a high-pressure tussle. The alternative response, as taught in judo, is to release such pressure by withholding force to create a downward momentum that can be used to throw an opponent with little effort. In this way, judo is about trying to use physics against someone, which is a handy skill in rugby league, as are the skills related to knowing how to fall and roll correctly.

Judo was helpful to Shane in several ways, and given he was at the dojo up to five times a week, he has never been a gym goer. All the strength and conditioning training he needs comes from time on the mat, and which just happens to be whole lot of fun!

There's no money in judo!

According to Shane, judo is run more as a sport than a business. Whilst some forms of martial art have become highly commercialised and branded – and driven by strategic business models – that's far less evident in judo. After having spent a decade at the top of the sport, followed by twice that amount of time running his judo school, Shane knows 'there's no money in judo'. It's something people do for the love of the sport, and for the benefit they get out of it – the competition, the camaraderie, the strength, the conditioning, and its other health benefits. But there's also something else Shane has valued about the sport – it's potential for inclusiveness.

This is something he came to appreciate a decade after retiring from competitive judo. After moving from Sydney to the NSW Central Coast, Shane was looking around for a place to have a wrestle. When he couldn't find a dojo that suited him, he decided to start his own club, and did it fairly quickly. After getting some gear together, and some interested people, he ran his first class in a school assembly hall. Soon, parents asked if he would run children's classes, and he did. Today, over 15 years later, the club has 130 members and Shane's teaching 20 times a week, with separate classes for different age groups, from very young children to teenagers and adults.

Opening up the dojo

Age wasn't the only thing that influenced the club decisions Shane made. He was also interested in opening the dojo to children with special needs, such as kids who were on the autism spectrum or living with cerebral palsy. At that time, judo wasn't being used as an activity option for cerebral palsy, but Shane knew it could be done – and done well – having seen it many times at dojos in the Netherlands. So, he started adding classes to his weekly program, and in so doing, began changing the face of his sport in Australia.

Although he experienced initial resistance to this change, Shane argued the case and people eventually saw the value. It was to give these kids options they had never had before. Kids who were usually confined to wheelchairs for sport were now out of their chairs and wrestling on the mat. In time, thanks to Shane's strong advocacy, the national association endorsed what he was doing, and now a special needs category must be included in every tournament.

Always pack your suit

Despite his whole-hearted involvement in the sport, judo has never been an occupation for Shane. He started out as a plumber, and became a sports administrator before becoming a schoolteacher. Throughout it all, judo has only ever been a sport for him. When he competed, he did it in his spare time and during his holidays. If he went on international trips, it was on the back of money he'd saved up, and on those occasions when he was in the UK, extra money he sometimes got for playing semi-professional rugby league.

One of the great things about all of his competition and travel – other than the sport – was that it helped Shane to develop an extensive national and international network of friends and acquaintances. Access to a community of like-minded people who shared his love of the sport and always welcomed others who shared that love. As such, Shane is always sure to pack his judo uniform before any trip. He likes the thought that he can go almost anywhere in the world, turn up to a dojo, and have a wrestle.

The benefit of an individual sport

In Shane's mind, everyone should be encouraged to do a team sport, for all the obvious reasons: the teamwork, the camaraderie, the challenge, and the enjoyment. That said, he thinks it's also important to feel the pressure of an individual sport, so participants can become more self-reliant, resilient, and confident. And in this regard, judo is excellent. He sees these benefits emerge, year after year. Countless children and adults who come to the dojo and learn how to look after themselves physically, learn how to roll and to fall, and learn how to control their strength and aggression, become more self-assured human beings as a result.

It's hard to overstate the importance of judo to Shane's life. It's given him so much, he can't imagine life without it. Thanks to that boy down the street all those years ago, Shane's living a highly active life, having a wrestle four times a week, and performing well against athletes half his age, which just shows that he's 'still got it'. And one thing's for sure: Shane doesn't intend to lose it. In the meantime, he's intent on doing everything he can to put his beloved sport 'on as many street corners as possible'.

Kayaking

What is it?

Like several other physical pursuits covered in this book, the word 'kayaking' can refer to many ways of recreating on water. This means there are many different types of kayaks, designed to suit whatever the aims of a paddler might be. For instance, there are different kayaks for paddling on flat water, white water, and sea water, surf ski kayaks for riding waves, and still others for those who want to fish, dive, do multi-day touring, or just have fun for a day. Whatever the purpose, the basics are the same. Kayaking involves sitting in a long, shallow, narrow, lightweight boat and propelling it through the water with a double-ended paddle. In some kayaks this is done by sitting *in* the boat, with the paddler's legs enclosed within the shell of the kayak, while in others it is done by sitting *on* the boat, with legs exposed. Ordinarily, kayaks are made of stiff fibreglass, but it is now possible to purchase inflatable and folding kayaks that have made transportation and storage much easier.

What are its origins?

The history of kayaking is intimately tied to the history of canoeing, with the latter predating the former. Canoe use stretches back almost 8,000 years and was relatively widespread. Early forms of canoe were used by the First Nations peoples of Australia, South American Indians, and other indigenous populations, and were usually made from hollowed-out tree trunks. It was an innovative use of natural resources to principally help with fishing and transportation.

Whilst canoe design benefitted from the evolution that occurred in boat building over many thousands of years, it was the colonisation of the world by European countries that drove further innovation. Most notably, this included using wooden frames and other light materials in their construction, making canoes lighter and more manœuvrable than row boats, and easier to use in the exploration of new territories. And it was from two such territories, far north Canada and Greenland, that the first kayaks are thought to have emerged. Developed by the Inuit tribes of those regions, kayaks were useful because they allowed individual hunters to move quickly and quietly whilst hunting seals, whales, fish, and other vital food sources.

As such, kayaks have a long history as working boats, and a much shorter history as leisure craft. The first reports of their recreational use come from Europe in the 19th century, followed by a steady increase in popularity that led to its inclusion in the 1936 Berlin Olympics. Like rowing, most competitive kayak racing takes place on a flat-water course, with events for one, two, or four paddlers (K1, K2, and K4 events). However, other kayak classes do exist. The most notable of these is white-water slalom racing, which has become an increasingly popular spectator sport.

What rules, if any, does it have?

Competitive kayak racing has a simple objective: to paddle a boat along a course in the fastest possible time. Despite the existence of several different classes of kayaking, the rules of the sport are relatively standard. Races occur between two points on a course of a pre-determined length. Beyond equipment changes that are specific to the class of kayak, the primary rules govern:

- Lane changing – boats must stay in their appointed lanes and not impede or obstruct other boats

- False starts – boats must not begin until the starter's gun fires, with two false starts leading to disqualification
- Results – finals usually consist of six qualified starters, with winning medals awarded in gold, silver, and bronze

The joy of it all

Kesley is a 40-year-old process improvement manager. He's been having fun in kayaks for about eight years and gets the most enjoyment from surf ski kayaking. His involvement in the sport started over 20 years ago, in the back of a two-person canoe, paddling down a river in his native South Africa. The event was the legendary Fish River Canoe Marathon, a challenging adventure race he was talked into by his best friend's father. Tall, athletic, and 18 years old at the time, Kesley seemed like the ideal choice to provide some horsepower at the back of the boat. As forward propulsion was his primary job, he was nicknamed 'The Motor'.

An intense introduction to paddling

Held over two days, the marathon travels roughly 80 km down the Groot-visrivier (Fish River), through rapids, over weirs, and across several land-based sections that require competitors to carry their canoes for hundreds of metres or more. This makes it a gruelling event, and it is not without its dangers. Over the history of the event, some of the challenging white-water sections have resulted in fatalities. Paddling Fish River twice proved an intense introduction to the sport. However, he did enjoy the way river paddling connected him to the natural world and helped to settle his mind. The changing scenery, the reeds and the rapids, the birdlife, the isolation, and the moments of peacefulness. As unique an experience as the canoe marathon had been, twice was quite enough! However, it did help him to discover some things about paddling that he very much liked. In time, he'd make a point to seek them out again.

After his Fish River experiences, Kesley didn't paddle again for quite a while. Instead, he turned his attention to other physical pursuits, like swimming, cycling, and running. He was also a regular gym goer and gave mixed martial arts a try for a few years. This is how Kesley likes to roll. He's a naturally active guy who likes to maintain a good level of physical fitness.

Finding a way to make it happen

In 2010, Kesley moved to Australia and settled in Newcastle, a large port city 180 km north of Sydney. It's situated on a beautiful stretch of coastline, with golden-sand beaches, prominent headlands, and a protected inner harbour. Not long after he arrived, he noticed that small groups of surf ski kayakers regularly paddled on the still waters of the inner harbour, and they seemed to be having a great time doing so, as he often heard them chatting and laughing as they cruised by. Having already had some paddling experience, this seemed like something he might enjoy too. So, he got to thinking…

Now, any sort of kayaking takes some effort to get started in. First and foremost, you need a boat. Then, when you get a boat, you need to be able to safely store it. But kayaks are quite long and awkwardly shaped, which makes storing them difficult. Then, when you have a boat and a place to store it, you need someone to paddle with. Surf ski kayaking is not without its risks, so having one or more paddle buddies is recommended.

For a newly arrived South African, these logistical and social challenges needed to be resolved. But wanting to make the most of this opportunity, he decided to join his local surf club. His initial reason for joining was to complete his Bronze Medallion, an Australian life-saving qualification, but Kesley had a bigger plan. He was looking for a way to get into paddling and realised the surf club was a great option, as they had plenty of kayaks. His plan worked perfectly. He got his Bronze Medallion, along with the start he wanted in paddling. But he also came to value the surf club so much that he become a beach patrol captain, and eventually Director of Surf Life Saving.

Paddle buddies

Soon after joining the club in 2014, Kesley became friends with Jordan and started paddling with him three times a week. These initial outings were limited to the flat, relatively still waters of the Hunter River, a short distance inland from the coast. But this was a crucial first step to take, because Kesley had never paddled a kayak, let alone a surf ski kayak.

At this stage it's worth explaining a little about the hierarchy of boats that are powered by paddles. Up to this stage, the only paddling Kesley had done was in a canoe, which is shorter and broader than a kayak. Canoes also tend to be open, with sides that give them depth and allow paddlers to sit inside. In contrast, kayaks are narrower, longer, and lighter. Most kayaks are designed for paddlers to sit inside, like canoes, but are not as deep as canoes, nor as stable. Then there are surf ski kayaks. As the name suggests, these kayaks are used in the ocean and designed with speed and manœuvrability in mind. It also makes them highly unstable and difficult to master.

Not surprisingly, all Kesley wanted to do on these early paddles was to stay on top of the boat. This required an incredible amount of persistence, and humility. After all, it can get a bit embarrassing – and physically tiring – to engage in a continual cycle of falling off and getting back on again. In Kesley's mind, this is the sport's major barrier to continuation – a test of resilience that self-selects for certain types of people, people who want similar things out of their recreation and are prepared to work hard for that.

A sensitive, sensation seeker

At this point you might wonder what sort of things was Kesley looking to get from his recreation? The short answer to that, using Kesley's words, is that it's about satisfying the 'sensitive, sensation-seeking side' of his personality. That's an answer that needs some explanation.

For Kesley, surf ski kayaking provides a chance to experience feelings of harmony via a sensitivity to the surrounding world. As challenging as his experiences on Fish River were, he also enjoyed moments of great peace and contentment. Moments where he was floating down the river, feeling a connectedness to the natural world he'd not felt before. It was a sense of communion he wanted more of, and surf ski kayaking offered a way to do that. But Kesley is also naturally adventurous and enjoys a good buzz – he has a thrill-seeking side to his personality that gets satisfied when he feels the surge of a wave under his boat, the radical unpredictability of it, the need to be fully focused, and to also be strong, balanced, skilful, and quick.

Clearly, Kesley feels a deep connection to his sport. At this point in his life, surf ski kayaking seems to be the fullest expression of himself. And it's spiritual. For him, paddling out through the waves is like going to church. He does it along with like-minded others (and the occasional dolphin or whale), but finds opportunities to be alone with his thoughts, process the events of his life, and make important decisions. Then, when he's finished doing all that, he can flop over and take a quick swim – a baptism, if you will!

The bond among paddlers

Jordan was Kesley's first paddling buddy, but it didn't take long before Kesley found himself part of a group of dedicated paddlers, people who persisted with the training process and were reaping the rewards, including improved balance and strength of character. People who felt that their sport had 'saved' them, for one reason or another, and given them a social network they could depend on. Positive people who loved a good coffee, a good laugh, and a detailed post-paddle debrief. It's something he just can't imagine being without these days, and he intends to continue with it for many years to come.

Luge

What is it?

Although luge is nothing like fencing as a sport, it's exactly like it in another way. How? Well, it's an Olympic sport, which means most of us don't think about luge except every four years, at which point, for about two weeks, we become utterly fascinated by it. It's a sport that, after a couple of days of binge watching, we've absorbed enough information – jargon, competitor profiles, basic technical knowledge – to speak with authority, should someone mention it at a family dinner or work function. Then, about a week after the Olympic cauldron has been snuffed out, all the information falls out of our head for another four years.

Luge is from the family of sliding sports that includes bobsleigh and skeleton. Like these sports, luge is not for the faint-hearted. However, you will already know this if, like us, you've watched run after run with your heart in your mouth, hoping the sliders get to the bottom in one piece. And that's the basic challenge. Luge athletes lie supine (face up) on a sled, before pushing off, feet first, from the top of icy track to get to the bottom in the fastest time possible. They can travel at speeds of up to 140 km/hour, using only their legs to steer. In case you missed it the first time, luge is not for the faint-hearted!

What are its origins?

The use of sleds is ancient and can be traced back 4,000 years to the Egyptians, who used them to transport cargo over sand.

However, sleds were more useful in colder climates, for the transportation of goods and supplies and, eventually, people. As a form of recreation, sledding dates back to 15th century Northern Europe, although it didn't become a competitive sport until the late 19th century. The latter was partially due to the efforts of a Swiss hotelier, Caspar Badrutt, who attracted customers to his St Moritz hotel with winter resort packages that included sledding.

As recreational sledding grew in popularity, delivery sleds were modified to increase their speed – early versions of the racing sleds now used by lugers. The first organised meeting of the sport took place in 1883, and in 1913 the International Sled Sports Federation was founded. Luge was introduced into the Olympics in 1964 and has been included in every Olympic Games since. Although traditionally dominated by German athletes, male and female, sliders from Austria and Italy have also achieved success.

What rules, if any, does it have?

The rules of luge apply uniformly across the sport, with no distinction made between elite performers and novices. In a competitive event, an athlete's time is the combined total of four separate runs, which are completed on the same track. The winner is the slider with the lowest combined time. In luge, athletes must:

- lie in a supine position, feet first
- wear helmets with face shields
- wear specialised boots to keep legs in a straight, compact position

Because of the high-risk nature of the sport, considerable effort is made to improve its safety, including continual enhancements to personal equipment and track layout.

The joy of it all

Alex is a 27-year-old professional luger who has represented Australia at the last three Winter Olympic Games (Sochi 2014, Pyeongchang 2018, Beijing 2022), and each time has improved on his previous performance (32nd, 27th, and 16th place, respectively.) Alex didn't discover luge until he was 15 years old. This was not surprising, as he grew up far north Queensland (Townsville), with little exposure to winter sports. His initial connection to the sport came after his mother encouraged him to attend an athlete recruitment weekend in Sydney.

As Alex was a highly active kid, athletic, and possessed a strong competitive streak, she thought he might find the sport intriguing, so they made the trip down. After being introduced to luge, and undergoing some athletic testing, it was decided he should go to the only place resembling a luge track in Australasia: a natural track near Queenstown, in New Zealand. After returning from Queenstown, Alex was keen to continue. And so he did.

A natural slider

Soon after, Alex took his first trip to the northern hemisphere, to the site of the 1980 Winter Olympics, Lake Placid, in New York. This was where he had his first genuine experience of luge on an ice track, confirming for him that (i) he liked the sport, and (ii) he had some talent for it. Soon after, others started to notice, and Alex received an offer to train with the Latvian national team. For an athlete from a non-luge country, this was a golden opportunity that he delightedly accepted. Over the next six years, he would live outside Australia for approximately eight months of each year, and spend four years with the Latvian team, a year with the US team, and a year with the International Luge Federation (FIL), a team of athletes from smaller luging countries with no national team. This prepared him for three Winter Olympics Games, numerous World Cups, and several other international events.

The thrills, the mechanics and the calm

Alex found luge an enjoyable sport right from the start. Most immediately, he found it appealed to the adventure-seeking side of his personality. This was especially the case in the first few years, when he was learning his craft and almost every run would be a thrilling experience. However, as he became more experienced and familiar with the major international tracks, the thrill factor diminished slightly. He still gets a thrill, certainly, but these days the biggest thrill tends to come with his first run at a track, beyond which there's the thrill of having a good run and recording a fast time. But there's a lot more to luging for Alex than just the thrill. And, interestingly, the enjoyment he gets from it has changed quite a lot over time.

One of the most enjoyable things about the sport for Alex is how precise it is. It's a precision that extends well beyond smoothly and accurately guiding a sled down a track. According to Alex, the mechanics of luging can really suck you in, mechanics that lugers need to know, such as becoming familiar with all the materials that make up a sled, how different types of steel influence speed on the track, and how to use track information to best calibrate a sled, such as the radius measurements from different bends. At times, this aspect of sliding has so captivated Alex that his coach has needed to redirect his focus from the sled itself to using the sled.

Regarding other sources of enjoyment, it might not come as a shock to learn that Alex likes doing well. By his own admission, he's a competitive guy, so he loves to compete. Understandably, he's proud of his Olympic achievements and his steady rate of improvement from Sochi to Pyeongchang to Beijing. Not bad for a guy who grew up in Townsville, where the only place to find ice is the kitchen freezer.

The quest for self-mastery

In the eight years Alex has been luging, his feelings for the sport have transitioned over time. In the past two years, that transition has been quite profound. And, unsurprisingly, the COVID-19 pandemic had a bit to do with that.

After achieving Australia's best result in luge at the 2018 Olympics, his good form continued into 2019. However, after returning home at the end of that season, he, like millions of others, found his life severely restricted by lockdown, particularly an inability to travel overseas. For an Australian in the sport of luge, this was hugely frustrating. With no access to a track or specialised training facilities, Alex was forced to halt training and competition for nearly a year and a half.

Paradoxically, this turned out to be a very good thing. At that stage in his career, he had been on the luge circuit for eight years, travelling constantly, always living in wintery environments, and accumulating all the aches and pains that come with being an elite athlete. His mental health was also a concern. Whilst he was flourishing on the track, he was starting to languish off it. So, in a very important way, lockdown worked for him. He needed a break, and he got it.

What luge can teach a guy

As Viktor Frankl once famously remarked, 'The greatest freedom we have is to choose our attitude', to choose what things mean to us. No one likes having their freedom restricted, but when life gives us lemons (like a lockdown), the only sensible choice is to make lemonade. At least, that was Alex's view. After dealing with the initial frustration of lockdown, it dawned on him that this presented an opportunity. He used the time to recover, allowing his body to do the healing it needed. And he started to read. Quite a lot as it turned out. On topics like mindfulness, which seemed relevant to succeeding in his sport, and to succeeding in life, more broadly.

Whilst it's tempting to conclude that luge athletes are 'adrenaline junkies', that's not quite right. Like anything, the more experience you have of something, such as sliding down a track at 140 km/

hour, the less it affects you. Indeed, strong emotions – positive or negative – are the last thing a luger wants. As Alex explains, when you're about to push off from the top of a luge run, what you need is a quiet mind, one that's supremely focused and ready to respond to whatever the next 60 seconds will bring.

This is much easier said than done. Alex needed time to learn the skills and embed the practices that could help. Lockdown gave him that chance. He established a regular meditation practice and worked out how to combine it with other forms of mental skills training, like visualisation. He was searching for a mix of practices, and by the time lockdown was over, he'd made good progress.

Looking forward to 2026

Olympic athletes tend to think in four-year blocks. Naturally, Alex is already thinking about Milano Cortina 2026, in Italy, the site of the next Winter Games. And what do you suppose is a key driver for him now? The refinement of his mental skills training practices. After coming out of lockdown and not sliding for 18 months, Alex was amazed to discover he was sliding better than he had been before the break. He puts that down, mostly, to improved mental health and better mental preparation. And after placing 16th in Beijing, he's not done yet, not by a long way. He wants to continue developing and honing his approach to see how much more it can enhance not just his performance on the track but also his life. He's intrigued by those possibilities and that luge offers him that.

So, there it is – luge. It might not be for everyone, but for Alex it provides huge satisfaction and enjoyment from the thrill he gets from sliding and competing, the fascination he has in its technical aspects, and the chances it gives him to develop greater self-mastery. All good reasons for him to stay connected to the sport for as long as he can.

Mountain Biking

What is it?

Mountain biking is an umbrella term used to describe the sport of riding bicycles off-road, across a variety of terrain. Whilst this often involves riding up and down mountains (known as 'all-mountain' or 'enduro' riding), mountain bikers have several variations to choose from. These include cross-country, downhill, four-cross, free-riding, dirt jumping, trail riding, mountain bike touring, bike packing, and its inner-city equivalent, urban bicycle motocross (BMX).

Mountain bikes share all the basic features of a standard road bike, however, design modifications such as shock absorbers, larger wheels, wider tyres, strong but light metal frames, and hydraulic disc brakes have all been necessary innovations to permit riding across rugged terrain. This has helped riders to access areas that were not previously accessible, but most mountain biking happens on clearly marked tracks and trails that are regularly maintained and easily found via published guides and maps. Importantly, these publications usually include easy to extreme trail-rating systems, which give both experienced and inexperienced riders the chance to plan their participation in the sport.

What are its origins?

The bicycle is a very modern invention, with the earliest designs first appearing in the early 19th century. A characteristic of these early bikes, like the penny-farthing, was that riders sat atop a large front wheel, placing them high off the ground. The major disadvantage of this design was that it gave riders a high centre of gravity and made them susceptible to toppling over, which restricted riding to flat, relatively even terrain. However, as bike design evolved and a rider's centre of gravity was lowered, the use of bikes on uneven ground became possible. By the late 19th century, this had progressed to a point where the US army had an Infantry Bicycle Corps.

Despite these early signs of a movement from on-road to off-road cycling, it wasn't until the second half of the 20th century that the origins of the sport can be seen. This was motivated, in part, by European road cyclists who were increasingly turning to off-road riding – cyclocross – as a way of keeping fit during the winter months. By the late 1960s, interest became more widespread across Europe and North America, and led to the emergence of the first custom-built lightweight bike designs. This further increased interest and participation in off-road cycling during the 1970s and eventually led to mountain biking becoming an Olympic sport in the 1996 Atlanta Summer Games, and included in every Summer Olympic Games since.

What rules, if any, does it have?

There are two reasons why it's hard to provide a concise overview of the rules of mountain biking. First, as mentioned above, there are many different forms of mountain biking, and each has variations regarding the equipment (e.g., frame and tyre size), and rules that govern competitive events. In addition, some forms of biking – like bike packing – are non-competitive and therefore not subject to rules per se. However, there are some important general principles to follow. As mountain bike design permits riders to access more and more remote areas, a degree of self-reliance is needed to ensure safety. This includes maintaining fitness levels required for the type of riding undertaken, appropriate trip planning, being well equipped (with maps, food, water, first aid, and tools), and having sufficient mechanical knowledge and skill to avoid becoming stranded when off-road (e.g., fixing flat tires).

The joy of it all

Vinnie is a 53-year-old executive chef. A proud New Zealander, he who grew up in the coastal city of Nelson, at the top end of the South Island. This is a picturesque part of the country, and an environment that encourages active living. For Vinnie, this meant lots of cycling, which included riding five kilometres to and from school each day, and a few years of road racing thrown in. It also included a lot of recreational riding with friends up and down the many river valleys and coastal plains of the area. Depending on how you choose to look at it, he was either fortunate or unfortunate enough to live in the hills that overlooked the city, which meant any ride from home would always end with a hill climb.

That sounds like fun!

As a result of these childhood experiences, Vinnie became quite adept at cycling. You could say he has a long history with road cycling, but that's not the case with mountain biking. In fact, he's only been riding off-road for two years and was 52 when he first sat on a proper mountain bike. This happened as part of a social event organised by his restaurant staff. They decided a day's mountain biking was in order, and Vinnie's interest was immediately triggered. He reckoned it sounded like a lot of fun, and given that he'd never ridden off-road before, it was something new. Off they went, for a day in the hills. Vinnie absolutely loved it.

The first thing he had to do that day was to get sized up for a bike. As he settled onto the seat, he was immediately struck by the differences between road bikes and mountain bikes. Of course, he already kind of knew this – he knew what a mountain bike looked like – but he'd not really had a close look at their shock absorbers, tyres, etc. Once he got going, he quickly discovered how it was that mountain bikers could do the things they do. For someone who'd only ridden road bikes, which have zero shock absorption, it was weird to ride a bike that could absorb the force of bumps and jumps, and effectively mould itself to the terrain. Although it felt odd, it also felt great. That first ride was 45 minutes, and after an initial period of adjustment, he found himself laughing most of the way down the track.

More opportunities for father-son time

With his childhood interest in cycling re-ignited, Vinnie quickly saw its possibilities. Almost immediately his 14-year-old son Jack took an interest. But mountain biking isn't the cheapest of sports. All those design modifications come with a cost, plus there's the need for car racks, home storage, and maintenance. Although this wasn't necessarily enough to stop him, it did give him reason to pause. If mountain biking was to become a regular physical pursuit, he needed to know he wasn't acting on a whim. Was it worth investing in the equipment? Would the initial spark of interest grow into a longer-lasting flame?

He didn't have long to wait for an answer. It came whilst holidaying with his family, near a national park that had good bushland and several mountain trails, setting mountain biking on the activity agenda, with the family deciding to hire some equipment and do some exploring. For Vinnie this was another great experience, and his boys really enjoyed it too. By the time they returned home, it was clear that mountain biking was worth pursuing. It was time to head to the bike shop.

Focus, forests and fitness

Vinnie is a busy guy. If you'll pardon the pun, running a fine dining restaurant is an all-consuming occupation, especially when you also service annual festivals and community events. As a result, his spare time fluctuates a fair bit, depending on restaurant commitments. This has tended to make mountain biking a once-a-week affair. But whenever he can dedicate time to a ride, he does.

There are several things he likes about the sport. First, he likes the intense focus it requires. In many ways, the concentration needed is not unlike that for alpine skiing and luge. As he describes it, if you want to successfully go from the top of a mountain bike track to the bottom, it's critical to be fully focused on what you're doing. You simply can't be off somewhere else in your head – you need to constantly process what's happening around you, calculating the steepness of a slope, the angle of a corner, and the positioning of your body on the bike.

Naturally, focused concentration is also critical to run a commercial kitchen well, but the challenges are very different, and there's little risk of Vinnie dislocating a shoulder while plating up an order. However, that possibility does exist when he's out riding on a trail, if he's not switched on, and it's an element of the sport that he really likes.

Another aspect of mountain biking that he likes is the immersion in nature. Being surrounded by mountains, forests, and rivers is something that reminds him a lot of his childhood experiences in New Zealand. It has also helped him feel an enhanced sense of gratitude about where he and his family live. Thirteen years ago, Vinnie and his wife, Jen, moved from Sydney to Hobart. They had a desire for a 'tree change'. It's a decision they've had no reason to regret, but Vinnie's mountain biking experiences have helped him to appreciate even more the value of that decision, helped him to see just how much they have gained.

Finally, it's been enjoyable to see the improvement to his physical fitness and sense of wellbeing. Whilst this might seem like an obvious statement to make, it's come with a couple of surprising twists. One was the realisation that he might enjoy his sport even more if he made a concerted effort to get fitter. So he did. A logical, if somewhat ironic place for a chef to start was with his diet. Running a restaurant is a stressful job and can lead to some less-than-healthy eating and drinking habits. But, armed with a good reason to improving his diet, Vinnie made some changes, kept up his physical activity levels, and quickly saw some positive results. Then – surprise, surprise – he found he had more energy when he was on the bike, and a greater capacity to do more.

Do I need a lift? Don't be ridiculous!

Vinnie's also come to realise just how much the cycling community can spur you on to greater things. Following a chance meeting with a cycling friend, just after Vinnie had ridden down a popular mountain track that overlooks Hobart, Vinnie shared where he'd been and casually mentioned that Jen had driven him up to the trail head, at the summit, earlier in the day. To Vinnie's surprise, this was greeted with a smirk and some laughter.

This was the moment he learnt about an unwritten rule of hardcore mountain bikers, which was that if you want to ride down a mountain, you must first ride up it (a bit like those early alpine skiers). This gave Vinnie pause. Should he? Could he? As it turned out, he proved more than capable of going all the way up before coming back down, and has successfully done so more than once. He's got there on the back of an improved diet, better body composition, and a determination to take up the challenge.

As far as Vinnie's concerned, mountain biking is very cool. It's allowed him to reconnect with a form of physical activity that he's always enjoyed and given him the chance to surprise himself, and at the tender age of 53, no less. It's also something he can do with his boys, engaging with the natural beauty of the place the family calls home. All in all, a great result!

Netball

What is it?

Netball is one of the few team sports to be included in this book. It also happens to have one of the highest community participation rates in Australia. One of the reasons for that is that it caters for all ages. For example, being low-contact, energetic, and social makes it a great starter sport for kids. It's also highly aerobic, skilful, and dynamic, which makes it engaging for adults. This makes any netball complex a very busy place on a Saturday morning, with numerous matches happening at once, something that continues into the afternoon as the junior matches finish and the senior and Masters matches start. But netball has also recently innovated to cater for much older adults and people with physical restrictions, with low-intensity 'walking netball' now an option. It's a good example of a sport breaking down barriers to participation.

Netball is played on a rectangular court, 30 metres long by 15 metres wide, which is divided into three playing zones: the attacking, centre, and defensive thirds. Games are played with a ball that is marginally smaller and lighter than a soccer ball, with the aim to score more goals than the opposition by passing (throwing) it down the court and shooting the ball through an elevated hoop at the end of the court. Of the seven players on a team, each has a specific attacking or defensive role, and can only move in the third(s) permitted for that position.

What are its origins?

Netball is an adaptation of basketball. When basketball was invented in the US in 1891, women were unable to play due to the imposed dress codes of the time. However, the new game quickly captured the attention of college teachers in the US and England. Several attempts were made to adapt a form of women's basketball, and an alternative game evolved that did not involve bouncing the ball and limited the court movement of some players. It is generally believed the first game of so-called netball took place in England in the late 1890s, but once established, it spread quickly throughout the British Empire and became popular in countries like Australia and New Zealand (where it was called 'women's basketball' until 1970).

Despite this growth in the game, it wasn't until 1960 that the rules were standardised. This happened when the sport's most prominent playing countries met to define a formal set of rules and formally establish the International Federation of Women's Basketball and Netball. This paved the way for the first World Championship to be held in 1963 (in Eastbourne, England) and much later for netball to make its debut at the 1998 Commonwealth Games in Kuala Lumpur.

What rules, if any, does it have?

As mentioned, netball is low contact. To be more accurate, it is defined as a 'contact contest' sport. This recognises that players striving for a ball naturally make some contact with each other, which makes it permissible. However, non-contest-related contact in netball is not permitted and is closely monitored during game play. Where an umpire deems unnatural contact to have been made, a free pass is awarded against the offending team. Other rules include:

- Position-based court restrictions – for example, a 'goal shooter' can only play in their attacking goal circle, whilst a 'wing defence' can play in the centre and defensive goal thirds, but not the defensive goal circle; such rules apply for every position, with the centre awarded the greatest freedom of movement
- Not holding the ball for more than three seconds
- The need to be three feet (90 cm) from opposing players in defensive situations

The joy of it all

Susan is 44 years old and the Chief People Officer of a large manufacturing company. She's also a netball nut. It's a game she's played almost continuously since the age of seven, paused only twice when pregnant with her two daughters. That's an impressive total of 34 seasons. Oddly, her netball life began because her brother played soccer. As it happened, all of the sisters of the boys soccer team members wanted to play something, but because soccer was not yet considered a sport for girls in 1985, netball was the obvious choice. This was also partly a matter of convenience, as it allowed parents to coordinate and take turns transporting the boys to soccer and the girls to netball.

Susan enjoyed it right from the start. It helped that she enjoyed some early success, with the team making the grand final in her very first year, a vivid memory for Susan. She was playing goalkeeper against a very tall goal shooter and remembers being told by her coach to defend against this girl in a specific way, whilst being given very different sideline advice from her father. Susan did her best and, to her absolute delight, the team won, followed by the 'best party ever'. She was hooked.

'Sticky' teammates

One of the things Susan cherishes most about netball is the lifelong friendships it's given her. She's been playing with a core group of friends – Alison, Vicki, and Toni – for the best part of 26 years, since Susan was 18 and they found themselves in a team together. Their connection was immediate and founded on a good mix of personalities, a sound understanding of the sport, and a shared interest in competing and doing well. For them, it created a relationship 'glue' that's seen them stick together for almost a quarter of a century.

But for Susan, there's more. She finds her friends hugely inspirational. All are at least five years her senior, yet they have remained incredibly fit and as enthusiastic and committed to the game as ever. The strength, speed, and endurance they show, week in, week out, motivates Susan. As she jokingly puts it, 'I want to be exactly like these women when I grow up'.

There's one other thing too. One of the main reasons the group has lasted this long is because of the psychological safety they've created for each other. What does that mean? It means that whilst they share a healthy desire to win and do well, they also share a cast-iron commitment to be open and honest with each other about the things that matter to the team and to each other. This makes them more than just a netball team. They're a close group of friends who share personal highs and lows without the fear of being judged, and with the certainty of support.

When the game fits, play it!

Aside from the social element, what does she love about the game itself? For one thing, she thinks the sport aligns well with her personality. Susan is a goal setter. She likes seeing how good processes (training) can lead to good outcomes (results), and netball gives her that. She likes focusing on competition matches and tournaments, and the game's many disciplines: footwork, passing cohesion, game strategy. And because netball is a game with lots of specific rules, especially around footwork and player contact, Susan finds it hugely satisfying when the team gets it right on the court.

This happened beautifully in 2014, when the team travelled to the Gold Coast to take part in the Pan-Pacific Games. They entered the Masters tournament and did well enough to make the semi-finals. Trailing by five goals at three-quarter time, the team rallied to tie the score by full time, before going on to win by two goals after extra time. Elation! It's one of Susan's most cherished memories – better, even, than her Under 10s championship win. There she was, battling away with her best friends, not expected to win, and getting the job done. Although they didn't go on to win the gold medal match, they took home a silver medal, and it meant an awful lot. Then, just to prove it wasn't a fluke, they repeated the result in 2016.

Spreading the love

Sport is an important part of Susan's life. It's a value she shares with her husband, Steve, who started playing soccer when he was four years old and has been playing for 53 consecutive seasons. As you might imagine, these interests have been a big part of their 20-plus-year relationship, with each supporting the other's goals. It's also a value they have instilled in both of their daughters who, thanks to Susan's encouragement and coaching, also developed a love of netball and have gone on to become representative players.

Motivated by a desire to spread her love of the game, Susan has coached quite a bit at junior level, an interesting experience, particularly over the last few years, because it's helped her understand what it is that she loves about the sport, which has shaped her coaching motto: 'Netball is a thinking sport'. It's something she tries to instil in her players, the belief that they can develop their game intelligence by thinking strategically and mastering its core skills. Beyond coaching, she's also been motivated to make a bigger contribution, as she knows that the sport relies on community volunteering. As such, she's taken on the role of Coordinator of Coaching at her local club.

A team is like an onion – it has layers

As you might imagine, Susan is rarely at home on a Saturday. Typically, you'll find her in the vicinity of a netball court, either doing something coaching related, umpiring, or playing herself. Whatever it is, she's involved somehow, just like many of her teammates – which is a handy segue back to the social side of the game.

As mentioned, Susan has a special connection her teammates. But we've not told the whole story. You see, there's another layer to the team, four more good friends who, thanks to Susan, joined the original group 10 years ago. This happened after Susan went off and played in a higher division for three years, a decision that Alison, Vicki, and Toni totally supported. As luck would have it, she went from one wonderful team to another and eventually got the idea that both sets of teammates should come together. Happily, everyone agreed and the original group of four were joined by Michelle, Karen, Carly, and Sue. Mixing social groups can be a tricky business, however, in this case, Susan's instincts were sound. The expanded team came together exactly as she'd hoped, and have been together ever since.

The importance of sticking together

Susan can't imagine her life without netball; it's just too important. Her teammates have become some of her closest friends and the bond is so strong they've gone to great lengths to remain a team. This was evident in the recent decision they made about dropping down a grade, because some of the older players were concerned they weren't quite matching the speed and energy of much younger opponents. Committed to staying together, they argued their case to the local association, who were admittedly reluctant to demote such an accomplished team. Happily, they got the approval and have continued to play, which is good because this team still has goals. Goals to play in Masters tournaments together, lots of them, including the World Masters Games. Goals to remain competitive, have as much fun as they can, and then, when the time does come, make a graceful transition to walking netball to keep the magic going.

Open-Water Swimming

What is it?

Open-water swimming takes place in naturally occurring bodies of water, like oceans, lakes, and rivers. This makes it ideally suited to swimming long distances, as swimmers can continue uninterrupted for sustained periods of time, without the frequent turning required in a standard 50- or 25-metre pool. As such, it is quite common for open-water swimmers to swim distances of up to 10 km, although much longer swimming challenges are regularly undertaken in many parts of the world. This includes the sport's 'Triple Crown': the English Channel (34 km), Catalina Island (32 km), and Manhattan Island (46 km).

Naturally, open-water swimmers encounter an array of challenges absent in swimming pools. For example, water visibility can sometimes be poor, because environmental conditions greatly affect how much a swimmer can see underwater, due to debris, mud, and/or the absence of sunlight. Relatedly, this can also make navigation a challenge, as ocean floors, riverbeds, and lake bottoms do not provide a conveniently painted straight black line. As such, to stay on course, an open-water swimmer needs to lift their head out of the water from time to time. In addition, open water is subject to tidal flows, currents, and swells, none of which occur in modern swimming pools. Finally, as open water is not the natural habitat of human beings, swimmers are aware that it is the natural habitat of other creatures, not all of which are necessarily friendly. All this means that open-water swimmers need to be ready for anything, and give some thought to what they are doing.

What are its origins?

Whilst swimming is not as natural a form of human movement as walking and running, there is evidence to suggest that some form of swimming existed in ancient Egypt over 2,500 years ago. Indeed, human survival has relied heavily on living around open bodies of water (e.g., fishing, transportation), so a basic level of water competence had to have existed. There is also evidence that swimming formed part of military training in ancient Greece and Rome, and was deemed to be important in the education of young men.

Recreational open-water swimming is a much more modern phenomenon. Typically, the origins of the sport are pinpointed to a swim undertaken by Lord Byron in Turkey, on 3 May 1810. On that day he completed several crossings of the Hellespont, part of the water passage several kilometres wide that separates Asia and Europe. Although his effort did not create a surge in the popularity of recreational swimming, by 1896 competitive swimming had become popular enough to warrant inclusion in the first modern Summer Olympic Games, in Athens. At that event the swimming events were held in the Bay of Zea, and after that an open-water sport continued for another two Olympics, with the 1900 Paris events held in the river Seine, and the 1904 St Louis events held in a man-made lake. Olympic swimming was first contested in a pool at the 1908 London Games.

What rules, if any, does it have?

Open-water swimming is a relatively straightforward sport, requiring little equipment beyond a swimming costume and a pair of goggles. Swimmers can choose to swim using any stroke they prefer; most opt for freestyle. Where rules do exist, they focus on two areas of concern:

- Drafting: This is prohibited in most events, with swimmers forbidden to swim closely alongside, or directly behind, another swimmer, preventing any advantage being gained from the reduced water resistance created by a lead swimmer's wake
- Wetsuits: Different events have different restrictions regarding the types of wetsuits that can be used; some wetsuits are designed to increase buoyancy and lessen water resistance, so these rules are applied to prevent swimmers from gaining an advantage based on something other than their swimming

The joy of it all

Kristen is a 39-year-old public servant who has had a love affair with swimming for over 30 years. Like most kids in Australia, Kristen learnt to swim at a very young age, and by the time she was eight, she was training with a swim squad and competing. Within 18 months she was the nine-year-old state breaststroke champion, which kicked off several years of success at both state and national levels. There was little doubt: the kid could swim.

After eight years of competitive pool swimming, Kristen stumbled across ocean swimming. When she was 16, she took part in an aquathon that was being held at a local beach. It was something different for her, a combined event that involved an ocean swim, followed by a run. It was her first experience of ocean swimming. She absolutely adored it and has never looked back.

A totally different experience!

When Kristen swam out through the breakers that morning, she knew only too well that her love of competitive swimming was waning. For years she'd been getting up at 4.30 a.m. to train before school, followed by more training after school. The sessions were typically very intense and focused on only one thing: speed, chasing target times and qualifying for events. Whilst she did enjoy doing well, over the years she increasingly disliked the process that supported her success. She was ripe for a change.

There were two things that Kristen immediately liked about ocean swimming. One was the sense of adventure she felt, and the other was a bigger feeling of achievement.

Regarding the adventure, the differences could not have been clearer. With a pair of goggles on, there is, quite literally, a world of difference between the clarified, predictable world of a chlorinated swimming pool and the varied, unpredictable world of a coastal shorefront. When swimming in the ocean, Kristen feels privileged to be there. It allows her to see gropers, stingrays, dolphins, turtles, and the occasional reef shark, as they swim under and across ocean shelves and in and out of sea caves. This means that no two swims are ever the same, and conveys a strong sense of adventure to her experiences.

Regarding achievement, Kristen finds the ocean infinitely more challenging than an Olympic pool. Pools are static environments, with a consistent water temperature, depth, and wave pattern. In contrast, the dynamics of the ocean bring extra dimensions of challenge. It requires her to deal with the constant shift of tidal flows, currents, and swells. In addition, whenever she's competing, there's the challenge of massed starts and trying to get underway without lane ropes to organise the field. This makes any ocean swim more of an achievement, something she often feels a great sense of pride over, and one that helps to keep her motivated.

Life goes better with swimming

For Kristen, swimming is an essential part of life. In any normal week, she'll swim at least four times a week, often as much as four kilometres at a time. That might sound like a lot, yet it's what gives her a sense of balance, and a feeling of being physically and mentally strong. Although she'd prefer to do most of her swimming in the ocean, oftentimes that's just not possible. For starters, she's a working mum, with a family schedule that doesn't always allow it. Added to that, the ocean isn't always suitable for swimming, because of bad weather, poor water quality, or occasional alerts about unfriendly marine life.

As a result, pool swimming remains a part of her life, but she doesn't mind that. Nowadays, she's focused far less on speed, so the pool is used to hone her fitness for the physical activity she loves the most. But during the COVID-19 lockdowns, with pools, gyms, and almost all organised sporting options shut down, Kristen was lucky to still have access to the ocean. Away from land, she was granted temporary relief from the pandemic, a place to decompress and clear her head, and immerse herself in the beautiful world that lies beneath the waves. This made her luckier than most during the lockdowns, and she knew it. More proof, in her mind, that life goes better with swimming.

Adventure, achievement – and ambition

When Kristen swapped the pool for the ocean 20-plus years ago, she did so because she wanted more from her sport. She wanted greater interest and enjoyment. It had become too narrowly focused on speed, and that just wasn't enough for her. Thankfully, she found the perfect alternative. However, it would be a mistake to conclude that Kristen had lost her competitive drive. She hadn't. As soon as she transitioned out of the pool, she started competing, and for someone with her competitive instincts, ocean swimming had plenty to offer. So, Kristen has always had a lot to focus her training on, along with a lot of ambition. For example, she would love to win her age category in events like the Cole Classic, in Sydney, and the Coolangatta Gold, in Queensland.

But beyond simple competition, she loves challenging herself and being bold. Like the time she and a friend went out and, on a whim, swam four and a half kilometres up and back along the NSW Central Coast. This was one of her COVID swims and one of the most memorable swims of her life. Everything about it was invigorating: the glorious weather, the crystal-clear water, and the sense of freedom – her version of a perfect day.

Days like that really spur her on and help to draw up a bucket list, a list of things she'd really like to do when the time is right, things her family would be able to enjoy with her. At the top of the list is crossing the legendary English Channel, closely followed by island swims in Fiji and Hawaii, and the Rottnest Channel Swim in Western Australia. It's an exciting agenda that fills her with excitement and possibility.

No 'bad' people

One of the things Kristen values most about ocean swimming is the people. For her, the sport is a great leveller. She likes that it takes people as they are – whatever their body shape, whatever their occupation or background, and whatever their fitness level. And she adores how the people are so encouraging of others.

In fact, she reckons that she's never met a 'bad' person on the beach. From her observation, the people in the ocean swimming community share a love of the ocean that creates an incredibly positive environment. Everyone is considered an equal, and everyone is interested in what others have done and what they might do. When people finish a race, the first question they get asked on the beach is not 'What time did you do?' The question is always 'How did you find it out there?' She loves that people share these stories with a camaraderie that's hard to beat.

An important part of the social side of her sport is safety. Kristen, like all ocean swimmers – is acutely aware that the sport has risks. But people make sure they always swim with others, they freely share information about when and where to swim (or not swim), they allow less experienced swimmers to wear extra gear (e.g., snorkels, slippers) so they can safely complete events, and no one leaves the beach until the last person has finished – and been given a massive round of applause. That's just the way that ocean swimmers do things.

Padel

What is it?

Padel is a ball sport that blends tennis with squash. Like tennis, matches are played on a court with a net, similar line markings, and slightly softer balls. However, unlike tennis, the court is enclosed by fibreglass walls, resembling a squash court. And like squash, players can keep the ball in play by hitting it off the side and back walls, using a variety of shots. The sport derives its name from the stringless bats that are used, generally perforated fibreglass, carbon fibre, or graphite. Whereas tennis and squash employ racquets that have strings, in padel the ball is struck with what can be best described as an over-sized table tennis bat.

Padel matches are typically played using a doubles format, with two players per side on a court that is 20 metres long and 10 metres wide. Singles matches are played on slightly smaller courts, six metres wide. In each, the presence of back and side walls means that the ball often stays in play for longer than tennis, and can give the game an intensity that is similar to squash. This makes it an exciting game to watch, where spectators are close to the action and have complete visibility.

What are its origins?

Padel is generally said to have been invented in 1969 by influential Mexican businessman Enrique Corcuera, but its origins are not quite as clear cut as that. Whilst the sport most obviously reflects tennis and squash, and is easiest to explain with reference to both, it should be noted that Corcuera had some historical models to guide his so-called invention. These include earlier sports such as 'real tennis', a form of indoor tennis dating from the 16th century and, most notably, 'platform tennis', an all-weather outdoor version of the game devised in the late 1920s.

In Corcuera's case, it was paddle tennis that inspired his effort to create a new ball sport at his home in Acapulco. Retaining many of the features of platform tennis, he innovated a court space with no out-of-bounds play areas, including the use of side and back walls, which would potentially keep the ball in play for longer. Having differentiated the game in this way, Corcuera played it with his many domestic and international visitors, who greatly enjoyed the game and helped to establish it in Spain and Argentina by the mid 1970s. Since that time, the sport has become very popular in Europe and South America, and has also spread to North America, parts of Asia, and (as you will shortly learn) Australia. According to some estimates, padel is one of the world's fastest-growing sports.

What rules, if any, does it have?

For anyone familiar with tennis or squash, the rules of padel are not difficult, as they are a faithful combination of both sports, including using the same scoring system as tennis, and permitting shots to be played off and onto the back and side walls, like squash. Rules specific to padel include:

- Only underhand serving is permitted
- If the score in any game reaches deuce, the normal tennis deuce rules apply; however, in professional tour events, a single 'golden point' is used to decide such games
- Players are permitted to leave the court (via open doorways on either side) to return any ball that goes over a wall

The joy of it all

Matt is a 39-year-old business owner with a long sporting history. He started playing tennis at the age of four, and rugby soon after. Playing both an individual and a team sport was clearly something that suited Matt, as he made tennis and rugby his summer and winter alternatives all the way through until he was 18 years old. Accomplished in both, Matt regularly ranked in the UK Top 10 for his age, whilst also trialling for the national team in rugby.

Despite Matt clearly having more sporting ability than most, his parents were both schoolteachers and concerned he retain a good balance between sport and study. After turning down a scholarship to play tennis in America, he decided to commit to his studies by going to university in Wales, where he was fortunate to continue to play rugby and tennis. That would prove fortuitous, because a few years later, fate stepped in.

The apple doesn't fall too far from the tree

When Matt was 21, he received an offer to work as a tennis coach in Spain. It came at a time when he was training hard, regularly competing, and trying his best to make a living from tennis. Although he'd never really considered himself a coach per se, the opportunity to be paid to play and coach seemed too good to turn down. He accepted, moved to Spain, and, in so doing, changed his life forever. Ironically, by becoming a professional coach, Matt had inadvertently begun to follow in his parents' footsteps, something he thought he'd never do. Admittedly this wasn't classroom teaching, but it meant drawing on a very similar skill set, one that Matt had some affinity for, through the modelling provided by his parents.

Living and working in Spain gave Matt the chance to experience padel for the first time. In Spain, padel is a very popular sport, with an estimated 20,000 courts and four million players. One of the reasons for its popularity is that it's a very social sport, and the way the Spanish play it, a whole lot of fun. Matt liked it immediately, partly because it closely resembled tennis, but mostly because it added several things tennis just didn't have.

A fun and lively sport

The more Matt became familiar with the sport, the more he understood why the Spanish liked it so much. First, it is a very social sport. Being primarily a doubles game, padel typically involves four players, whereas it is more common in tennis to play singles, with only two opponents on the court. Given that two padel courts take up roughly as much space as one full-sized tennis court, that translates to a player-to-court ratio of approximately 4:1. How does this make it more social? Easy. As games are played on smaller courts, the players are physically closer, and the game is more interactive. Then, when you factor in the Spanish fondness for having a good time, with music, tapas, and drink, an afternoon or evening at the padel courts becomes more like attending a social club.

But Matt was attracted to more than just the vibrant atmosphere that surrounded padel in Spain He was also attracted to the diversity of skills the game requires. Although he had never played squash before, the option of playing off the walls appealed to him, as did the way the sport encouraged him to play shots that he was discouraged to play in tennis, such as drop shots and lobs. This added a lot of interest and enjoyment for Matt and gave him the chance to play more creatively than he ever had before. As such, it was only a matter of time before he started to play competitively.

Opportunity came knocking again

Two years after starting to play, Matt found himself playing in Mexico at the 2002 World Championships. He was part of the first team to represent Great Britain in the sport, a team made up of four ex-tennis players. Their first elite level tournament was not overly successful, but then they hadn't expected it to be. Their goal was to gain more experience, and the World Championships gave them that. In the end, they came in 15th out of 16 countries, and in the process, achieved Great Britain's first international win (2–1, against Canada). Matt continued playing, however, the team had some disappointing results during the 2006 qualifiers and didn't make the main draw for the next World Championships.

Despite this disappointment, Matt had not only established himself as a competitive padel player but he was coaching now, as well. He also became extremely interested in growing the game in England and started looking for investors. By 2012, his plans had come to fruition and resulted in the establishment of the first padel-only club in the UK. These were Matt's first efforts to expand the game globally, something he would continue a few years later, on the other side of the world.

Padelling down under

Within the space of a decade, Matt had evolved from competitive tennis player and coach to (i) competitive padel player, (ii) tennis and padel coach, and (iii) sports entrepreneur. The more he got involved, the more he sensed the potential of the game, and the more eager he was to introduce it to others. So, when he was asked in 2015 to move to Australia and help launch the game, he didn't need a whole lot of convincing. Sensing a great opportunity to do something positive and exciting, Matt sold his padel club in England and headed down under.

Naturally, two of the main challenges setting up new padel courts is space and cost. But this is where Matt's long history with tennis has proven helpful. He knows how tennis centres work. He knows they tend to possess a lot of space because standard tennis courts are about 260 square metres, which converts to quite a bit of real estate when six or eight courts are involved. He also knows that those courts are not always used, and that padel, by virtue of its four-fold player-to-court ratio, offers an interesting alternative for tennis centres to maximise their primary asset. And this is how he and his business partner approached it. So far, it's gone very well and six centres have now been established: two in Sydney, two in Perth, one on the Gold Coast, and one in Melbourne. Their goal? Twenty-five padel clubs.

Building a legacy

For Matt, his padel project is significant for two reasons. First, he has always enjoyed his involvement in sport and gained a lot of satisfaction from coaching others and helping them to enjoy it. Second, he's an aspirational guy, someone who's always on the lookout for opportunities. Through padel, he's found an opportunity that is ideally suited to him: a chance to increase community participation in physical activity, leave a positive mark on the world, and help to future-proof both of the sports that inspired it.

For tennis, padel provides an interesting alternative to the core sport that, like T20 cricket, provides lots of thrills and an exciting atmosphere. For squash, padel may help to slow or even pause its more recent steady decline. Participation rates in squash have fallen for years, with many squash courts either repurposed as gyms or demolished. The growth of padel also helps to keep squash skills alive, whilst creating – using clear glass walls and a larger ball – a better appreciation of those skills by spectators.

Matt's excited about the sport, and excited about its future. And it's not just him. Word is spreading, and thanks to the presence of a show court at the 2022 Australian Open, awareness is growing. The future looks bright indeed for this hybrid sport.

Quadball

What is it?

Quadball is the sport originally known as Quidditch, a free-running ball game inspired by the *Harry Potter* book series. Whilst the game played by the wizard was air-borne and involved broomsticks, the ground-based version has been modified to account for gravity yet preserve as much of the fictional game as possible. Quadball is played on a rectangular field, roughly the size of two basketball courts. Like football or basketball, the aim is to score more points than the opposition, by throwing a partially inflated volleyball (the 'quaffle') through any one of three hoops positioned at either end of the field, yielding 10 points.

Of the seven players that make up a quadball team, each plays very specific attacking and defensive roles. During game play, all players are mounted on a one-metre-long wooden broomstick and, like dodgeball, they can be temporarily knocked out of the game if an opponent hits them with another ball called a 'bludger'. When this happens, the player who has been hit must retreat to their own hoops before tapping back in. The game proceeds like this for 18 minutes, at which time the 'snitch' enters the field of play, wearing a tag on the back of their shorts. Each team's 'seeker' attempts to end the game by catching the snitch and grabbing the tag, which is worth 30 points. Both sides' points are tallied to determine the winner.

What are its origins?

Not surprisingly, the original form of quadball was developed by fans of the *Harry Potter* series. It has its origins in the United States in 2005, when two Vermont college students devised the earliest version of the game and called it Quidditch. After some rule development, the game quickly spread across college campuses and soon was added to the list of team sports at several American schools, including the University of California. Further expansion of the game saw the establishment of a US national tournament in 2007, and by 2012 the International Quidditch Association (IQA) held its inaugural World Cup event. Quadball is now played in more than 25 countries around the world, making it a truly international game.

There is a temptation – because of the *Harry Potter* connection – to see quadball as a bit of a fad and a quaint storybook game that surely couldn't count as a real sport. But if you're tempted to take that view, we urge you to take a closer look. The people who play quadball are very serious about their sport. Indeed, the sport's foundational documents include the 160-page IQA Rulebook, which standardises how the game is played around the world and has been translated into six languages. In addition, rule amendments are also published, along with changelogs that reflect the evolving nature of the game. More locally, game play in Australia is directed in accordance with published policies on gameplay, injury, concussion, first aid, and extreme heat.

When you take a closer look at quadball, you see a sport that is well-organised, constantly evolving, and comes complete with five-year strategic plans. As such, it seems anything but a fad and, instead, destined to be around for many years to come.

What rules, if any, does it have?

The rulebook for quadball is very extensive and detailed, which is both a blessing and a curse. It's a blessing because there are few grey areas in the game, with rule updates meticulously recorded, and a curse because such an extensive set of rules needs to be administered, in real time, by a team of referees who need to remember all the rules. Rather than attempt to summarise all of its rules, we've opted to highlight a couple of the game's key features.

First, quadball is a full contact sport. As the aim of the game is to score more points than the opposing team, players are permitted to prevent attacking plays in a few different ways. One way is through body contact, which pp. 69–71 of the *IQA Rulebook* stipulates can be via body blocking, pushing, charging, and wrapping. If these contact rules are violated in any way, referees can award guilty players a blue, yellow, or red card. Is this what happens in a quaint storybook game? Probably not. If you're not keen on body contact, this might not be the game for you.

Second, quadball is also an all-gender sport. This is a very important aspect of the game, as it means that teams can be made up of cis (male or female), trans, non-binary, or any combination of genders. This rule is applied by only permitting four members of the same gender to be on the field at the same time. By not running the sport with conventional male and female teams, the game can be considered socially progressive. That is, gender inclusiveness sits at the heart of quadball, as does the creation of an environment that fosters a spirit of fair, robust competition for anyone who feels they can hold their own on the pitch. These foundations appear to have been key to the expansion of the game, and also a primary reason behind the name change, following an increasing desire to distance the game from the *Harry Potter* series.

The joy of it all

Alise is a 30-year-old mathematician and science communicator. She is also a lover of quadball. Her introduction to the game was slightly unusual in that she was an organiser of the game before she ever played it. Perhaps it would be more accurate to say that she needed to become a local organiser before she could become a player. We should explain…

If you build it, they may come!

When Alise was nearing the end of her mathematics degree on Queensland's Sunshine Coast, a friend showed her a YouTube clip of quadball being played on a US college campus. She was immediately intrigued. Not a naturally sporty person, she found the dynamic nature of the game attractive. Quadball is fast-paced, complicated, and often chaotic. Being mathematically minded, this appealed to her: the strategy, the complexity, the patterns. But the origin of the game was also appealing; she loved the *Harry Potter* books and that was, as for so many others, an immediate hook.

At the time Alise first learnt about the game, she wasn't very involved in the university's clubs and societies scene. As nothing much interested to her, she and a few friends struck on the idea of starting their own quadball team. This presented a slight problem, however, because quadball equipment isn't widely available. They had to start from scratch and get some equipment together. Whilst some things could be bought and modified, such as volleyballs, others had to be made (e.g., goal hoops and broomsticks). They got resourceful and before too long had enough equipment to facilitate a game, with enough people to play it. A club had been born!

All that happened back in 2014. Alise has been playing ever since, feeling no desire to stop after she'd finished her degree. These days she feels a bit like a veteran. She's gained a lot of experience, collected some war wounds (three broken bones), travelled quite a bit (to play, organise, or spectate), and become well connected across the sport. She's even, along with some teammates, had a quadball-inspired design tattooed on her ankle. Now, that's not the sort of thing you do on a whim; it's something you do when you're passionate about your sport.

So, what it is about quadball that Alise loves so much? Well, there are many things. Some of those are related to the game itself, and some are related to the culture that surrounds the sport.

The sport

As mentioned earlier, Alise is a mathematician and attracted by the dynamic nature of the game. Unlike other ball sports, where the focus of play is often centred on the position of the ball, in quadball there can be multiple focal points, as there are four balls in play at any one time: one main ball (the quaffle) and three additional balls (bludgers) that can temporarily remove other players from the game. As a result, it can often seem like there are three games happening within the same game, which means it's never boring.

Perhaps more than anything, Alise enjoys playing the role of a beater in quadball. The job of a beater is to be as disruptive to the opposition as possible – to spoil opposition plays, remove opponents (with accurate bludger throws), and generally engage in as much chaos-making as possible. She revels in it. Maybe, in a counterintuitive way, that reveals something of the mathematician in her. Perhaps when you spend a lot of time solving problems and resolving formulas, you delight in the chance to create problems on the field and leave other people to solve them? Whatever the reason(s), she gets a real kick out of it.

Another element of the game that she enjoys is how reliant it is on teamwork. Because of the game's complexity, it's hard to do well at quadball if you're not communicating well and working closely together. All of the teams Alise has played with tend to be quite closely knit and stick together over time, probably the reason, she says, she's played for eight years straight, longer than almost anything else she's ever done. That leads to the other thing that she loves about the game: its cultural aspects.

The culture

With each passing year, quadball has less and less to do with the *Harry Potter* stories. One way is through rule changes, which have been implemented to make the game more playable. The evolution of the game is also driven by limitations that exist because of the licenced ownership film studios have over words like Quidditch and quaffle, and other key terms, making it difficult to leverage commercial opportunities to expand and develop the game. However, as national associations adopt the name quadball, the sport will have more control over its own destiny.

Although these changes make the sport less like the game described in the *Harry Potter* stories, Alise isn't concerned. Yes, she loves the books, and those she plays with also love the books, but an increasing number of people playing quadball have never read a *Harry Potter* story. So, with each passing year, a fondness for *Harry Potter* becomes increasingly less important as the glue that holds the game together.

For Alise, one of the things that's become far more important is the culture of gender equality that has grown up around the game. She loves the fact that, as a relatively new sport, quadball is not hampered by a set of traditions that people feel tense about breaking. Rather, the people who play and run the game are actively creating a culture, one that welcomes everyone and creates an environment where people can be 'comfortable being their authentic selves'. She likes that it attracts a lot of interesting people, like-minded individuals who are progressive and committed to breaking down barriers amid a fun, competitive environment where personal identity is deeply respected.

For Alise, these are things she's always wanted to be a part of, and wants to stay connected to. A dynamic, challenging game with a bit of rough and tumble, and a culture defined by social inclusion and personal acceptance. That just goes to show a physical pursuit can sometimes mean a whole lot more than the mere physical activity itself. Brooms up!

Rowing

What is it?

Rowing can be an essential means of transportation, a leisurely form of recreation, or a vigorous competitive sport. As a competitive sport, rowing has the same basic aim as kayaking and canoeing: to propel a lightweight boat, known as a shell, along a course in the fastest possible time. However, rowing is unlike kayaking and canoeing in two important ways. First, rowers move forward by pulling their oars through the water, which is most efficiently done by facing away from the direction they are heading, whereas kayakers and canoers face forward. Second, in rowing, the oars are attached to the boat by oarlocks; in kayaking and canoeing the paddles are not connected to the boats.

To row well, rowers need good concentration, sound technique, and considerable mental and physical strength. They also need good coordination, especially when rowing with others, as they need to synchronise with other crew members. Races occur between two points on a course of a pre-determined length (e.g., 1,000 metres), with the winner being the crew to cover the distance in the least amount of time. Over the years, variety has been added to the sport through the addition of boats that can be crewed by one, two, four, or eight rowers. In some cases, the larger boats (fours and eights) are allocated a coxswain, whose job it is to steer the boat and coach the crew through the race.

What are its origins?

Rowing, like running, swimming, and surfing, has a very long history. From the time humans used boats to travel on water, paddles and oars would have been a key form of propulsion. Whilst the evidence of vessels being rowed for transportation dates back more than 4,000 years, the first evidence of it having a competitive focus is much more recent. For example, funerary carvings for Pharoah Amenhotep II (ca. 1430 BC) indicate he was a capable rower, and the ancient Greek storyteller Virgil describes competitive rowing as being included in the funerary games of that time.

Given the prominent place rowing has occupied in the lives of people through the ages, it's not surprising that rowing is one of the earliest forms of organised sport. The oldest, continuously held rowing race is the Doggett's Coat and Badge race in London, which was first held in 1715 and has run annually ever since. As an organised sport, rowing gained prominence in the mid 18th century, when it became a focus of intercollegiate sports for several prestigious universities and colleges in the UK and US. By 1900, its status as a major sport was confirmed when rowing made its debut at the Paris Olympic Games.

What rules, if any, does it have?

Despite the existence of several different classes of rowing, the rules of the sport are relatively standard. Beyond equipment changes that are specific to the class of boat, the major rules relate to:

- Lane changing – boats must stay in their appointed lanes and not impede or obstruct other boats
- False starts – boats must not leave the starting line until the starter's gun fires, with two false starts leading to a disqualification
- Results – finals usually consist of six qualified starters, with winning medals awarded in gold, silver, and bronze

The joy of it all

Zoe is a 27-year-old psychology student. Although a little older than most undergraduate students, there's a good reason for that. You see, until recently, Zoe was a full-time athlete. She rowed for New Zealand and did very well. A multiple national and international titleholder, she won World Championship gold in the lightweight single sculls (2015, 2016), and in the lightweight double sculls (2019).

Zoe loves rowing, but it hasn't always loved her back. As in boxing, lightweight rowers face the constant pressure of having to 'make weight' before they compete. For five years, Zoe accepted this pressure as the cost of competing at the highest level. In time, however, the cost became too great. Her physical and mental health were badly impacted, so much so that Zoe made the only decision she felt she could make: four months before the Tokyo Olympics, she retired from the sport she loved. In doing so, she stepped away from the very real possibility of an Olympic gold medal. By prioritising personal health over personal glory, Zoe took the road less travelled. It's a decision she insists she has never come to regret.

Back at the beginning

Zoe was 13 the first time she climbed into a boat, followed, almost immediately, by another first, falling out of it. Truth be told, falling out of boats was something that Zoe had a real talent for. So great was her talent that she got the *Best Swimmer* award from her teammates in her first season. It was not an award she would permit herself to win again.

A little context is important here. The setting for Zoe's introduction to the sport was Otago Harbour, in Dunedin, the capital of New Zealand's deep south. If you've ever been to Dunedin, you know it can be a very cold place, and not known for its aquatic sports. It takes a hardy, determined person to put up with a regular dunking in Otago Harbour. It just so happened that 13-year-old Zoe was just such a person, which is why she never gave up.

At this point, you might be wondering why a girl living in chilly Dunedin would choose rowing. Good question. Zoe had shown some talent for netball and been an interprovincial 800-metre runner, so she did have options. Zoe's fascination with rowing was triggered, though, during the 2008 Beijing Olympics. Like the rest of the country at the time, she was enthralled by the exploits of her countrywomen, Georgina and Caroline Evers-Swindell, identical twin sisters attempting the sport's first-ever Olympic title defence. Zoe vividly remembers watching the final, the tension of the photo finish, and the ultimate elation generated by their victory.

She also remembers being captivated by the look of the sport. She liked the beauty of the movement, the boat gliding across the water, the twins working in unison and flowing as one. But Zoe couldn't quite make sense of what she was seeing. How were they were making it all happen? She wasn't sure. That race planted a seed in Zoe's mind, and as it turned out, it wasn't long before she'd start answering her own questions.

Learning together

Zoe got started in rowing through school. After attending a meeting about the sport, she was keen on it, but shy and nervous. Luckily, her mum, Trudy, worked at the school. Fearful that her daughter might miss an opportunity, to Zoe's great embarrassment she pulled her out of class to attend the first team session. As it turned out, this was a team Zoe was always going to make. Not only had none of the kids had ever rowed before but the coach already had Zoe pencilled in to make up a new pairs crew.

At this point, Zoe's determination became crucial. Rowing is a challenging sport to get started in, and staying upright and balanced is the first major challenge. This was initially part of what motivated and interested Zoe: she wanted to prove to herself that she could do it, and she wanted to make sure she wasn't bad at it. Fortunately, she was in a team of rookies, so everyone made plenty of mistakes, and there was lots of laughing and learning together.

These were Zoe's initial steps on a journey that would eventually lead to the top of her sport, a journey that would result in World Championship medals, national recognition, and, very nearly, to the Olympics. But let's get back to what she has loved about it.

'A bubble under your boat'

Rowing is a precision sport. To move a boat through the water at optimal speed requires good balance, good coordination, and good timing, physical and mental challenges that remain the same, whether you're a world champion or an amateur club rower. These were challenges Zoe always loved to try and conquer. Challenges like perfecting the entry of her blades into the water, so that the oars would 'catch' well and allow maximum force production. Challenges like building boat speed in a race and being so synchronised and smooth that you feel there's a 'bubble under the boat'. Challenges like developing trust with your crew mate, and learning to rely on each other, as you pull for their success and they pull for yours.

In a way, by engaging with these challenges, Zoe was answering some of the questions that first arose whilst she watched that 2008 Olympic final. Answering through the experiences she had, like those of the Evers-Swindell twins, of working in unison with another. Rare moments of optimal functioning – what psychologists call 'flow' – where difficult challenges are met by well-ingrained skills. Peak experiences where time really does fly, when you know you had fun and the satisfaction is huge.

But, wait, there's more!

Aside from her fascination with the physical, psychological, and social sides of rowing, Zoe loved the connection it engendered with the surrounding world. Most treasured of all were the sunrises – hundreds of them – usually enjoyed from the middle of a lake, and often enhanced by encounters with such marine life as fish, dolphins, and sea lions.

But, mostly, Zoe's on-the-water training sessions made life simpler. With no technology or others to distract her, these sessions gave her a single point of focus and were stress-free and enjoyable. They provided opportunities for deep connection with her training partners, where she could share the things that were on her mind and be there to listen in return. Some days, she says, these conversations were like 'therapy session on water', and an important part of team bonding, building understanding and trust within the boat.

Life after rowing

Like many retired athletes, Zoe now finds herself in an unusual situation. Although her decision to quit competitive rowing was made for very good reasons, it also removed from her life a strong sense of purpose. To be clear, she still loves rowing. In time, she expects that she'll continue with it. But her challenge now is to work out how she can do that absent the strong sense of purpose that kept her going for a decade: the desire to become a better, faster athlete.

Not only is this unusual for her; it's also just plain unusual. When it comes to physical activity, most people struggle to generate the commitment they need to keep them moving. But Zoe has an extraordinary capacity to commit, along with an expectation that she will, but just not in the way she once did. And so goes life. The constant need to adjust and readjust. Amid reflecting on her successful rowing career, her studies in psychology, and her occasional forays onto the water, a compelling purpose is certain to emerge. Something that transforms what the sport means to her and allows her to forge a new relationship with it.

Surfing

What is it?

Surfing is a surface water sport where a specially designed fibreglass board is used to ride the face of a moving wave of water. Typically, this happens at sea- or ocean-facing beaches, although the right weather conditions occasionally make surfing possible in some lakes and rivers. In recent years, the emergence of wave technologies has seen the development of wave pools, generating opportunities for wave riding within commercial fun parks and even on cruise ships.

There are numerous ways to wave surf, and various sub-disciplines have been inspired by wave surfing. Surfing waves in a conventional way is done using a variety of different-sized boards, which range from short, light, highly manœuvrable boards (ideal for competitive surfing) to longer, heavier, and more stable boards (ideal for just having fun). A lot of surfing takes place at metropolitan city beaches, but the sport has become progressively more adventure-based, and it is common for surfers to travel to isolated areas searching for 'good breaks' or pursue 'big-wave surfing' with the aid of motorised surf skis. Other surf sports include windsurfing, kitesurfing, wakeboarding, and skimboarding.

What are its origins?

According to Matt Warshaw's encyclopædic *The History of Surfing*, the sport has a long and rich history. As he explains, some form of surfing has probably existed ever since man first started interacting with ocean waves. He backs this up by reviewing archaeological evidence of life in ancient Peruvian communities, and the likelihood that the small, flexible reed boats they used for fishing – *cabalittos* – may have also been used for recreational purposes. Some have disputed this, but few dispute that the Polynesian people of the Pacific were keen wave riders. Indeed, it appears they placed a considerable amount of social significance upon it, with the best wave riders often gaining high social status. According to historians, Polynesian surfing was happening as early as the 1700s, eventually spreading to North America in the early 1900s and becoming a popular global sport across the 20th century.

Today, surfing is one of the fastest growing sports in the world. According to the World Surfing Association, an estimated 50 million people surf worldwide. Some propose the reason is because surfing gives people an enhanced awareness and appreciation of the natural world, and may be related to the growing global concern about environmental issues. For others, an increase in surfing merely reflects the in-built attraction that human beings have for blue space (water), as a place to both experience a sense of calm and enjoy time with others.

What rules, if any, does it have?

The rules of many sports are often quite straightforward, but that's not the case in surfing. Here, there are both formal rules and informal rules. Formal rules are those that apply in a competitive event, dictating what entrants can or cannot do; for example, an event's permissible board size; the time allocated to riders in a heat; the way points are allocated to individual wave rides; and regulations about turn taking and not interfering with others' ability to catch waves. Informal rules are those that could apply at a beach anywhere in the world and are more like surfing etiquette, such as the expectation that riders will be supportive to other riders; visitors are to be respectful to the regular riders at local beaches; and that riders should be considerate and not 'drop in' on other riders if they have already begun to ride a wave.

The joy of it all

Kristen is 52 years old and works as a manager in a healthcare company. While many surfers start riding waves when they're quite young, Kristen didn't start until just after her 40th birthday. So, a bit of a late starter. Although surfing isn't her only form of regular physical activity, it's the thing she loves the most. She finds it more than a little addictive, and admits to getting 'edgy' if she's not been in the water for a few days.

You'd be forgiven for thinking these might be the reflections of a person who has lived by the ocean all their life. That's not Kristen. She grew up in rural New South Wales, a long way from the nearest beach. But because the family farm had a swimming pool, she spent a lot of time in the water and was a confident swimmer from an early age. Her mother insisted that her kids were capable around water, because of the rivers, creeks, and dams on or near their property. When Kristen moved to Sydney to go to university, she already had an affinity for the water, just no inclination (yet) to start surfing. That would take another 20 years.

Surfboats, Bali and the gift that keeps on giving

During her twenties, Kristen did what many people do in their twenties: she studied a bit, partied a lot, finished her degree, worked for a while, partied some more, and in the middle of all that, headed overseas for three years of fun and adventure. Basically, she had a great time. She swam, cycled, hiked, and ran – without settling on anything specific. That came when she was 35, when she got into surf boat racing. This was a different sort of physical challenge for Kristen, and one she really enjoyed. It was also a team sport, something she hadn't tried her hand at before.

Yet, as much as she enjoyed it, after five years spent competing in surf carnivals, it was time to do something else. That something else was surfing. She treated herself to a spot on a Bali surfing retreat and started learning to surf at the tender age of 40.

'I can't teach commitment'

Upon returning home, Kristen made a commitment to continue with it. She bought a 10-lesson program, secured a coach, and started working on her technique. It was during this period that Blake, her coach, gave her a piece of advice that she's never forgotten. He told her, 'Kristen, I can't teach commitment'. It was a message about being courageous and trusting herself. It was a message he felt she needed to hear, due to the tentativeness she displayed when catching waves, which is a sure way to get hurt, he told her. The way Kristen sees it, that advice wasn't just useful for surfing; it's proved to be a great metaphor for life, and a consistent point of reflection for her.

With Blake's help, it wasn't long before Kristen was committing to waves, getting better results and enjoying herself more. When that happened, she was able to enjoy even more things about the sport that have made it addictive.

Blue mind

One of the things she loves most about surfing is the deep connection it gives her to the ocean. She's not unique in this. A large body of research evidence shows that human beings have an instinctual connection to 'blue spaces', and that time spent near and around bodies of water (oceans, lakes, river, waterfalls) are beneficial to physical and mental health. This has certainly been Kristen's experience. When she's sitting 'out the back', watching the swell and waiting for waves, the ocean starts to weave its magic. She finds it soothing. The swell of the ocean has a regularity that's captivating, a repetitive pattern that differs just enough to never be boring. She's also found it enormously reassuring. After Kristen's mother died several years ago, she found that time spent in the surf gave her solace and a spiritual connection to her mother.

Kristen finds surfing to be a profound form of physical activity, providing her with a source of great challenge as well as a source of great comfort. But there are still other reasons why she loves it.

Meteorological mastery

She notes that it's virtually impossible to be a regular surfer and not pay attention to the weather. Tides, currents, wind direction and strength, swell, and storm cells – they all matter. They not only influence *if* you'll go looking for waves but *where* you'll go looking for waves. In the 12 years she's been a surfer, Kristen has become a keen observer of the weather, and as a result, developed a kind of meteorological intelligence she has come to rely upon. In fact, she's learnt so much about it that her friends often consult her when they have questions about the weather or want an updated forecast. That's just fine with her. Learning something while you're having fun? For a lifelong learner like Kristen, that's the icing on an already awesome cake.

'Surfing's like the mafia'

The social connectivity of surfing is another thing she loves. Kristen recalled a quote from surfing legend Kelly Slater: 'Surfing is like the mafia. Once you're in, you're in. There's no getting out,' speaking about a solidarity that exists amongst surfers. Something akin to membership in a club that attracts members from all walks of life and has little concern for someone's social status. Kristen loves that surfing has allowed her to connect with a range of interesting people that she otherwise might never meet.

She loves that the sport is a great leveller. The ocean doesn't care where you were born, what you do for a job, or how much money you have. And neither do most surfers. When you're sitting on a board in a wetsuit, no one's much interested in what happens back on land. You're out there with a common interest and a passion that's shared. Something gets into your blood and stays there. And that's true even when you pick the sport up a little later in life.

A sport for all ages

It would be easy to think of surfing as a young person's sport. But Kristen's story proves that you can pick it up later in life, learn a challenging new skill, and develop the level of commitment required. And you can compete. Kristen knows this because, recently, at age 52, for the first time she got to the final of a surfing competition. There she was, standing on the podium, feeling the warm glow of satisfaction. Getting a tangible reward for something that's always been intrinsically rewarding. A sport that's given her the chance to hang out with dolphins, to see stunning sunrises and sunsets, to go adventuring in Sri Lanka or Bali, and to share it all with people who only care about what you're doing now, not what you've done in the past, or currently do for a living.

There's something else about this that should be noted. Kristen was 40 when she decided to go to Bali and learn how to surf. This clearly shows that her decisions weren't being constrained by self-limiting beliefs based on her age. She wasn't looking at surfing and thinking, *nah, I'm too old for that*. She wasn't engaging in any *self-directed ageism*.

Rather, Kristen saw something she really wanted to do and said to herself: *Why not?* Then off she went and made it happen, uncovering a passion that she's been enjoying for well over a decade now. Given the positive impact surfing has had on her physical, mental, and social wellbeing, Kristen ranks it as one of the best decisions of her life, and one she'll always be thankful she made.

Table Tennis

What is it?

To state the obvious, table tennis is a version of tennis played on a table. To make it work as a game, everything was made smaller – the playing surface, line markings, net, balls, and bats. In almost every respect the game resembles its bigger cousin, except for a simplified scoring system that has players alternate the serve after every two points (although even that mirrors the tiebreak system in tennis) and requires a player to win by at least two points, once they have scored 11, 15, or 21 points, depending on which playing system is used.

Table tennis is one of the highest participation sports globally, and one of the most inclusive. Part of the reason for that is its simplicity. A game of table tennis is easy to set up, and the equipment is relatively inexpensive. Indeed, table-tennis tables are often found in family homes, and in a variety of recreational, educational, and other public facilities (e.g., holiday parks). This often makes it one of the first sports encountered by children, and because it is easy on the joints and is rarely traumatic, can be enjoyed by people across the lifespan. It is also a highly beneficial form of physical activity. Amongst other things, table tennis is known to enhance visual acuity, hand–eye coordination, improve reflexes, balance, and coordination, and provides an excellent form of brain stimulation whilst burning calories and providing opportunities for social connection.

What are its origins?

Table tennis has its origins in England. The earliest version of the game emerged as an after-dinner parlour game played amongst well-to-do members of Victorian society. It was played on the floor, using champagne corks as balls, cigar boxes as bats, and piles of books as a net. As such, the activity was little more than a distraction for the English aristocracy. However, as it grew in popularity, a series of innovations helped create the sport we know today. In 1890, Englishman David Foster introduced the use of a table. Then James Gibb went to the US in 1901 and stumbled across a light, novelty celluloid ball that seemed ideal. Soon after that, EC Goode introduced a hard, rubber-coated bat to the game, and the sport was set to flourish.

Originally, the sport was called ping-pong, due to the sound the celluloid balls made during play. However, the use of the name became restricted by a trademark owned by Parker Brothers, a US toy and game manufacturer, which forced many newly formed sports bodies to become Table Tennis Associations. Despite this, the game quickly grew in popularity. In 1926, the English and International Table Tennis Associations were formed, and the first official World Championships were held in London. By the 1930s the sport had become very popular in Asia, and continued to spread around the world. In 1988 it was given full medal status at the Seoul Olympics.

What rules, if any, does it have?

As mentioned, the rules of table tennis are very similar to those of tennis. That is, players play matches over three or five sets, with the diagonal service of the ball called a 'fault' if it fails to cross the net, and a 'let' if it touches the net during flight. Also, like a tennis tiebreak, players typically alternate the serve every two points, although some play variations have a change of serve after every five points. Other rules that apply include:

- The server must keep the ball in plain sight of the opponent and referee prior to serving
- To be a legal serve, the ball can only bounce once before crossing the net, and a legal return must be hit by the receiver before it bounces twice
- Neither player is allowed to touch the net assembly, or any part of the table, during play

The joy of it all

Peter is 70 years old and a retired public servant. He's been playing table tennis almost continually since 1974. He's only had two years off, between 2014 and 2016. These were two difficult years that saw him recovering from a stroke, an intercranial hæmorrhage that required him to be put into a medically induced coma for two weeks, then a physical rehabilitation unit for eight weeks, followed by months and months of hard work trying to rebuild his life. A highly competitive A-grade player in his prime, the hemiplegia caused by the stroke left him with paralysis in his right arm and leg. This was not only a challenge for day-to-day living, it was also a problem for his table tennis, because Peter was a right-handed player.

The greatest game in the world

According to Peter, table tennis is the greatest game in the world. This was his view before his stroke, but these days he is utterly convinced of it. In his mind, the game saved his life. Saved it by helping him to keep going. It helped him to stay active, both in body and mind. But we should go back a bit. When you've played a sport for almost 50 years, your enjoyment of it cannot be tied to one life event, no matter how catastrophic that might have been.

Peter first picked up a bat when he was 22 years old, which you could say was relatively late. Up until then, he was a soccer player, and a pretty good one. But this had to change when he started wearing glasses, as he couldn't comfortably head the ball. So, he looked around for something else to do and noticed that the local War Memorial Club held weekly table tennis nights. He started going, and played socially for the first 12 months. He took to it straight away and, eventually, a friend of his convinced him to start playing competitively. Being up for a challenge, Peter agreed and proceeded to jump right in at the deep end, playing A-grade.

A passion for the sport

When Peter started playing A-grade, he had a coach. But being coached, he says, didn't stop him from 'getting my bum handed to me on a plate each week'. Whilst it was a tough initiation, Peter kept at it, and as his game got better, he developed a reputation for being a bit of a swashbuckling player. A guy who plays the game hard and is confident enough to hit low percentage shots whenever he felt the need. In fact, this was so much part of Peter's game that he became known as 'hero', a player who was prepared to attempt shots others wouldn't normally try.

After playing for 10 years, Peter became more involved with the sport. He could see that things needed to be done to improve what was happening locally, and so he put together a submission for a sport grant, got it approved, and with it his club bought five new tables. This is the kind of thing he does, no matter where he plays. Peter has a can-do attitude, a deep love for his sport, and is always interested in helping others to share the love. Good equipment, he says, makes that easier.

So, what's so great about table tennis?

There are many things Peter enjoys about table tennis. One is the speed of the game. Despite the light balls, table tennis is one of the fastest ball sports in the world and it challenges him to remain alert and switched on. He also likes the strategy of the game – particularly doubles – where matches are like a game of chess:

trying to avoid your opponent's strengths whilst exploiting their weaknesses. He also likes the many ways it's possible to hit a ball. From a technique standpoint, that's given him lots to practice – hitting the ball with topspin, slice, or simply hitting flat and fast.

But he also likes what the game gives him physically and mentally. When he was a public servant, his matches were important, because he sat a lot during the day, and playing or practicing gave him some physical relief at the end of the day, as well as a solid cardio workout. Although it may not look like it, table tennis can really get your blood pumping, especially when you play like Peter. Another notable benefit is what it's done for him mentally. When you play enough, table tennis really sharpens your reaction times and visual system. This is something that Peter has confirmed every time his has an eye exam. He has good spatial awareness and excellent peripheral vision. There's no doubt in his mind that table tennis is responsible for that.

The game that just keeps on giving –

In Peter's mind, table tennis people are some of the best people. Over the years he's really enjoyed the camaraderie that comes with the social side of the sport. This was never better demonstrated than in 2016 when, after two years of battling his way back from suffering a stroke, some of his table-tennis friends decided to organised it so he could start practicing again. This suited Peter just fine, because being a non-playing spectator was excruciating for him. They set up a table and got him to do basic drills, lots of them, hitting hundreds of balls a session, with his friends there to gather them up and keep him going. This was the best rehabilitation imaginable, but also the toughest, because his hemiplegia had left him with little movement down his right side. As such, Peter was learning how to play with his left hand, and learning how to move a body with restricted movement. But he was determined to do it, all with the help of his friends.

– and keeps saving his life!

At this point, it's worth revealing that we both know Peter. We met him in 2018, two years after he started playing again. At that stage, he was doing remarkably well. Although his mobility was still restricted, he was playing competitively, in C-grade. At that time, his serve was unique. He did it one-handed, holding the bat and ball in his left hand, because he couldn't use his right. It was inspiring to see. His life might have been saying 'no', but Peter was saying 'yes'!

That's why, when it came to write this chapter, only one person came to mind. But we hadn't seen him in four years, so we weren't sure if he was still playing. Not only is he still playing, but when we arrived to interview him, a fit-looking Peter greeted us with a firm handshake – with his right hand! Naturally, this was something we were curious about.

As we chatted, Peter's statement that 'Table tennis saved my life' took on greater meaning. In his mind, there's no doubt that continuing with table tennis has driven improvements in his physical function. Although still restricted, his movement is much better. This is something people comment on all the time, and we noticed immediately. Apparently, he can toss the ball with his right hand now and, although he's still playing C-grade, the 'hero' still has ambitions. Perhaps most tellingly, Peter told us that when playing left-handed, he no longer has to think about what he's doing. Such is the plasticity of the brain – it rewires itself to allow Peter to play the sport he loves the most. A sport that has given him so much, and that he cannot imagine being without.

Footnote from Riley:

Table tennis is well known within the Spence household and some competitive father–son rivalry exists. Never was this more obvious than one weekend during lockdown in 2021. After some friendly trash-talking, a challenge was agreed: the first player to 1,000 points wins (provided they win by two points). Dad and I fought it out over several sessions across two days. The result? 1,000 to 996, in Dad's favour. That translates to almost 2,000 points over 7 hours of play! Personally, as much as I like the game, this challenge is not something I'd recommend, not unless you're really stuck for something to do. Also, it's worth being a bit strategic. Letting the old fella win has at least kept me clothed, fed, and sheltered…

Ultimate

Ultimate is a non-contact sport played with a flying disc. As a sport, it resembles American football in that the aim is to pass (throw) the disc down a field into an end zone to score points, and the team with the most points wins. Matches are played outdoors on a field that is 37 metres wide and 100 metres long, which includes a 64-metre central playing zone, and two 18-metre end zones. A point is scored whenever an attacking player successfully catches the disc mid-air from within the end zone. A game is usually won by the first team to reach 17 points, although the point limit can be negotiated prior to the start of play. Ultimate games usually consist of two 15-minute halves, with a five-minute half-time break.

Many people refer to the sport as 'ultimate frisbee', however, that's not technically correct. Ultimate can be played with any brand of flying disc that meets the size and weight specifications of the World Flying Disc Federation (WFDF). Frisbee is the best-known brand of flying disc, simply because it was the first.

Many sports in this book can be legitimately traced back thousands of years. Yet, although the ancient Greeks were throwing disc-like objects as early as the 8th century BC, no line can be drawn between the ancient sport of discus and the modern sport of ultimate. Indeed, the first versions of the game emerged in the early 20th century in a surprising way, courtesy of a group of US college students from Connecticut, who started playing flying disc games with discarded pie pans. They found that when the pans were thrown horizontally with a spinning motion, they flew rather well. This became part of the student culture for decades, as did the custom of calling out the name of the company that made the pies: the Frisbie Pie Company.

By the 1950s and '60s, the pastime had become so popular that plastic flying discs were mass produced, with the Pluto Platter, the Wham-O, and eventually the Frisbee finding their way onto college campuses. As the popularity of flying discs continued to grow, the emergence of a sport seemed inevitable. This happened towards the end of the 1960s, when students in New Jersey and Massachusetts developed a team game they called Ultimate Frisbee. In 1970, the first edition of the rules was published, followed later that year by the first competitive game, and in 1975 the first organised tournament. Once established, the sport spread quickly across the US and on to Canada, Japan, and numerous other countries. Today, ultimate is played by an estimated seven million players in more than 50 countries.

What rules, if any, does it have?

In ultimate, rules are enforced by adherence to 'the spirit of the game', which is akin to an honour code amongst players. This allows games to be self-refereed, with players accepting responsibility for fair play, rule compliance, and respectful conduct. It also means that opposing players must find ways to quickly resolve on-field issues related to rules, so the game can keep flowing. As for the rules themselves, here are a few of the basics:

- Only seven players are allowed per team
- Players are not allowed to run with the disc, but can throw it in any direction

- Throwers have a maximum of 10 seconds to throw the disc, whilst the closest defender counts the time (called a 'stall count')
- No physical contact of any kind is allowed between players

The joy of it all

Craig is a 47-year-old IT consultant who's been throwing discs for just on 30 years. He took it up in high school, back in South Carolina, when he needed to choose a sport to participate in. He had tried several different sports like cross-country running and basketball, but he and his friends enjoyed ultimate the most. They stuck with it until they finished high school and continued playing at college, where it was known primarily as a sport for geeks and hippies. This was of little concern to Craig, as he was concerned only with doing things he enjoyed, an enjoyment that has lasted for three decades and shows no signs of diminishing. There are several reasons for that.

Work out and geek out

Craig has always been an active person. Whilst ultimate is a competitive game which can be played to an elite level, he's never focused much on that. For him, the sport is a great way to keep fit, and he does that by playing a couple of times a week, doing some gym work, and running occasionally. But he also finds ultimate an interesting sport, interesting because ultimate offers throwing and catching possibilities that aren't available in other sports that use projectiles, such as American football, netball, basketball, and rugby.

According to Craig, someone can really 'geek out' on the physics and geometry of ultimate. This is because flying discs can be thrown in ways that aren't possible in other sports. For example, when preparing to throw a disc, the thrower can launch it on an almost infinite number of flightpaths by angling it in different ways, and by varying its speed and height at the point of release. This gives players a lot of scope to innovate and experiment with a core element of the game. In addition, the shape of a flying disc makes the game quite dynamic, as discs can be easily caught using just two or three fingers, rather than requiring the whole hand, which results in a lot of acrobatic, one-handed catching.

For Craig, the unique aerodynamics of flying discs make game strategy another point of interest. This relates to the challenge of reading the game and trying to choose the right throw at the right time: trying to anticipate player movements, visualise alternative plays, make quick decisions on the run, and then successfully execute passes whilst under defensive pressure.

The spirit of the game

Craig enjoys ultimate for all the reasons stated, but there's also a philosophical foundation of the game that he greatly values, called 'spirit of the game'. According to the WFDF, this is similar to the idea of fair play but with added importance. As stated in the rules of the game:

> 'Highly competitive play is encouraged, but should never sacrifice the mutual respect between players, adherence to the agreed-upon rules of the game, or the basic joy of play.'

Examples of 'good spirit' include informing players if you think you have caused a foul or made an incorrect call, complimenting an opponent for good play, introducing yourself to opponents, and reacting calmly to any disagreements that might emerge during game play.

The spirit of the game allows ultimate to be played without the need for a referee. Craig really likes this, because the sport is not hampered by an overarching 'hatred of the referee' that exists in many other sports. As such, ultimate precedes without this unhelpful source of distraction. That allows both a greater focus on the game itself and – importantly –shows faith in the players to adjudicate their own behaviour and conduct, along with the maturity to prioritise the good of the game over their competitive instincts and ego.

A source of disappointment

Despite being fundamental to the sport, good spirit has not kept the game free from officialdom. Whilst self-refereeing is still the norm across most levels of the game, the use of observers (to assist with on-field decision making) has become more widespread, and referees are often used in professional tournaments. From Craig's perspective, these are disappointing developments. Whilst he enjoys the competitive aspects of the game, Craig continues to see it solely as a *game*, and therefore appropriate for self-refereeing. Because of this, Craig prefers not to play in competitive games with observers and referees, opting for the more informally organised games easily found in many major cities.

Meetup.com

In a reflection of its college campus origins, ultimate continues to have a strong accept-all-comers community orientation, making it relatively easy to find a game of ultimate in most major cities around the world, which are often organised via Meetup.com, a social media platform for coordinating social events and gatherings. This keeps things simple, with game organisers able to announce game details – date, place, and time – in an easily accessible public forum. In Craig's experience, the use of Meetup and other social media platforms has helped to increase player diversity. Although the game still tends to attract university-educated players in their thirties and forties (often with engineering and IT backgrounds), over the past few years he has noticed a change in player demographics, both in age and occupational status.

The spirit of the game also underpins the acceptance and inclusion of all comers, irrespective of ability. Admittedly, that might not result in everyone being admitted to every game, as it depends on player turn out and skill levels, most ultimate players encourage participation. In Craig's case, this includes giving novice players impromptu lessons and, wherever possible, including them in games to help with skill development.

Another way the game has built participation and interest is through different game formats, such as 5-aside, mixed, and kids matches. Inclusion has also been supported via the use of 'hat' tournaments, where interested players put their name into a hat and are randomly drawn to join a team.

Making bigger contributions

These days, Craig's involvement exists on two levels, as both a player and an organiser. As a player he wants to keep playing for as long as he can. Although his knees aren't as good as they once were, his involvement has been prolonged by only playing in less physically demanding social matches. As an organiser, Craig has a goal to increase community awareness of the game and applies for grant funds to increase its outreach. In this way, ultimate is a lot like parkrun. That is, it's a community-based physical activity that can be easily organised, is focused on inclusiveness, and has virtually no cost. As such, its prospects for expansion seem bright.

As Craig explained, it is not unusual for those in the ultimate community to look for ways to make bigger contributions to the world. One such example is the Ultimate Peace project, which uses the game to build bridges to friendship, trust, and leadership between Israeli-Arab, Israeli-Jewish, and Palestinian youth. The project revolves around youth camps, where kids come together to live, eat, and interact. Given the deep social and religious disconnect that exists between these communities, it is hoped that by playing ultimate and adhering to the spirit of the game, children will both enjoy each other's company AND develop skills needed to resolve differences with people of diverse backgrounds.

Craig sees ultimate as more than just an enjoyable game. He values its philosophy and sees its potential to positively influence individuals and their communities. And that's reason enough to stay involved, even after his knees tell him he needs to stop playing ultimate and start playing disc golf.

Vigoro

What is it?

Vigoro is arguably a hybrid sport, because the original form of the game combined elements of cricket and tennis, but the game has since evolved into more of a fusion of cricket and baseball. As a game, vigoro more closely mirrors cricket, as competing teams attempt to score more runs than their opposition, using similar equipment (long handled bats, stumps), scoring protocols (the 4- and 6-run boundary system) and rules (methods of batting dismissal). Whether the invention of the game was an attempt to convert tennis into a team sport or create a more accessible form of cricket, no one is quite sure, but vigoro has stood the test of time – but only just. Once popular in the Eastern states of Australia, especially New South Wales, Queensland, and Tasmania, the 21st century has seen a decline in participation rates and a contraction of the game almost exclusively to Queensland. But the game does live on, with a socially inclusive strategic plan and continued hope for a revival.

What are its origins?

Vigoro was invented by Englishman John George Grant in 1901, a time when cricket and racquet sports like real tennis, lawn tennis, and squash were hugely popular in the UK. Keen to create a new ball sport, Grant took inspiration from these games and designed some new equipment and a new set of rules. First played competitively in October 1902 at Lord's Cricket Ground in

London, vigoro attracted some initial interest but never became popular in England. However, in the aftermath of World War I, the game found a home in Australia and quickly flourished. This was in no small way due to the passion and advocacy of administrators like Ettie Dodge, who was President of the NSW Women's Vigoro Association from 1919 to 1966, and the All Australian Association from 1932 to 1966.

A significant event in the history of vigoro was its adoption into the NSW school curriculum, as this introduced the game to children and greatly increased public awareness of the sport. As a result, participation rates increased steadily in the Eastern states of Australia and reached a peak in the 1950s and 1960s. Although not originally designed to be a game specifically for women, the original equipment and rule innovations made the sport appealing to women and were a key reason for its popularity.

What rules, if any, does it have?

The easiest way to understand vigoro is to make the obvious comparison with cricket and note some major differences. For example, in vigoro –

- there are 12 players per side, instead of 11
- games have time limits and rarely last more than two hours, less than the shortest forms of cricket
- only two players are allowed to bowl at any one time, with one using a red ball and the other using a white ball; unlike cricket, these are thrown, overarm, in an alternating colour sequence
- the game moves at a faster pace than cricket because both bowlers throw from the same end of the pitch, so the fielding side spends minimal time making positional changes; like baseball, this means that batters always hit from the same place

- batters must run anytime a ball is hit in front of the crease line, reminiscent of the 'tip and run' rule used in backyard cricket, increasing the pace of the game

The joy of it all

Deanne is a 49-year-old community resources officer. She started playing vigoro at school when she was 10, which was a year or two earlier than most girls. Having played quite a bit of backyard cricket with her father and brother, she was attracted to the game and thought she'd do well at it. So, she started to play, and 38 years later, she's still playing. As such, vigoro has been a very significant part of her life – and not just as a player. Following Ettie Dodge's fine example, Deanne is also a prominent administrator, President of her local club and the regional association.

So, what is it that she loves about vigoro? As it turns out, there's quite a bit.

Lots of ticks in lots of boxes

One of the things Deanne likes about the game is, well, the game. Thanks to her father and brother, she developed an early interest in bat and ball sports through playing cricket, which is *the* bat and ball sport of Australia. Fortunately, her dad was a pretty good coach and he taught her many of the basic skills in their backyard. But Deanne is also a self-starter and enjoyed training herself, which included using that classic Australian batting drill of repeatedly hitting a tennis ball pushed into a sock, as it dangled from the washing line.

When the chance came to play a bat and ball sport at school, she was in! Unfortunately, in the mid-1980s cricket was predominantly seen as a game for boys and not widely available to girls. But vigoro was still part of the school curriculum and Deanne was naturally drawn to it. When a friend said she also wanted to give it a go, the decision was made. They started playing, and she enjoyed it so much, she played all through primary and secondary school and participated in many interschool competitions.

An elegant simplicity

In Deanne's mind, vigoro has an elegant simplicity to it. As a player and an administrator, she's always liked how accessible the game is, both in terms of how it is played and the playing skills required. Being a faster form of cricket, vigoro has the effect of neutralising the most common criticism of the parent game – that cricket is so-o-o boring! Cricket traditionalists may not like it, but vigoro cuts a lot of 'dead time' by having bowlers bowl from the same end, which means that, unlike cricket, the game does not pause for two or three minutes after every six balls for bowling and fielding changes, and bowlers do not have time-consuming run-ups. Perhaps more than anything, vigoro gets its name (an Anglo-Norman word for 'vigorous') from a hit-and-run batting rule that keeps the game moving and all players on their toes.

It also has lower barriers to participation. According to Deanne, vigoro is not an overly complicated game, which makes it quicker to learn. An important part of this is the simplified bowling action that's used. Why does this create a lower barrier to participation? Simple. The conventional bowling action in cricket is hugely challenging. It involves running in, leaping, and rotating, mid stride, into a sideways position whilst simultaneously using the arms to bowl a ball down the pitch using a windmill action. This is a complex coordinative challenge that often takes children many years to master. Vigoro completely removes this challenge by permitting any throwing action that starts above the shoulders. This creates a reduced skill requirement and potentially makes it attractive to many more potential players. This is further assisted by the fact that it uses less equipment, as the softer balls eliminate the need for batting pads and helmets. As such, players can play the game very much as they are, with little need to fiddle around with or buy equipment. This also makes vigoro an inexpensive game to play.

A tale of two Deannes

When you talk to Deanne about her love of the game, you hear both the player and the administrator speak. You hear the sportswoman, the part of her that really enjoys friendly competition and has spent time playing soccer, golf, tennis, and indoor cricket. But you also hear the administrator, the part of her that cares about participation rates and the potential enjoyment that others could get from vigoro.

This is what makes vigoro a bit more than just a game for her. It's a channel through which she can make a positive contribution to her community by encouraging others to get out, get active, and, in so doing, create better connected communities. On that point, Deanne also likes that vigoro is a game that people can easily reconnect with. In her 38-year playing career, she's seen many women, including herself, pause playing while they have children or take care of life matters and then make a quick return to the game.

Amid all these positives, Deanne is acutely aware that the game is, from a participation standpoint at least, in decline. Over the last 25 years, the sporting landscape has changed a great deal and it's become harder and harder to retain players, let alone attract new players to the sport. But no one is giving up, and there are some things about the game that stand out.

A mixed, inclusive, multi-generational game

Deanne was recently pleased to be able to play with her daughter for the first time – and in the same team! This is not uncommon in vigoro. Indeed, there have been many examples of teams made up of grandparents, parents, children, aunts, uncles, cousins, etc., all playing together. There's even been at least one example of a girlfriend and boyfriend playing together. Yes, that's right, a male vigoro player!! That's not too surprising, as it turns out. In a development that would warm the hearts of the sport's founders, male participation in vigoro is being encouraged through the promotion of mixed teams. And more is being done to attract the involvement of members of the indigenous community through the organisation of First Nations rounds and carnivals. With these expansions, vigoro may also start to become more attractive to children and adults as a steppingstone on the way to cricket and other balls sports.

It's mainly about community

Anyone who knows about vigoro will tell you that it reached its high-water mark in the 1950s and '60s, and has been on the wane ever since. Indeed, Deanne and others who play the sport often wonder if people will still be playing it in 10 years' time. We hope they are. In a world where social disconnection and physical inactivity are all too common, the loss of a sport like vigoro would be disappointing.

According to Deanne, the vigoro community she's a part of is hugely important to the lives of many people. The social bonds formed during the friendly, relaxed atmosphere of vigoro matches continually pays dividends when times turn tough. Like the support that people have received during droughts, floods, and other natural disasters. Or when women have needed a safe space to go, for some positive interactions and a friendly ear. Or such as the hour or two that carers need to lose themselves in a game and get some respite from their responsibilities.

These are the things that drive Deanne. She has a lifelong love of the game and a desire to positively impact the lives of others. This is what has shaped her motto as an administrator: 'Do it with quality. Do it well. Offer people something beyond the sport.' In other words, give them a place to come to laugh, and a place to cry. Just make it real and the rest will look after itself.

Wheelchair Rugby

What is it?

Wheelchair rugby is a Paralympic sport played by men and women with significant physical impairments. The sport combines elements of basketball, handball, and hockey, but the game is identified as a variation of rugby because of the wheelchair collisions that regularly occur between players. This gives the game a rough and tumble look, as the chair-on-chair contact often results in players being tipped over and having to right themselves again. As such, it is not a game for the faint-hearted. It's also why the game was originally called murder ball.

Like rugby, the aim is to pass and carry a ball from one end of the court to the other, and score goals by running the ball over the opposition's goal line. The game is played on a basketball court and, like basketball, wheelchair rugby matches have four quarters, each lasting eight minutes. The winner is the team who scores the most goals at the end of the fourth quarter. If the score is tied, a three-minute overtime period is added and, if the score is still tied, further overtime periods are added, until one team wins.

What are its origins?

Wheelchair rugby was invented in 1976 in Winnipeg, Canada. It was originally designed to be an alternative to wheelchair basketball and provide quadriplegics with an additional exercise option. Although its growth was initially slow, by 1982 the game was being played in the United States and Australia, and in 1993 the International Wheelchair Rugby Federation (IWRF) was founded. This was also the year that wheelchair rugby became officially recognised as a sport.

After the IWRF was established, the growth of the sport became more rapid, with the first World Championships held in Switzerland, in 1995, followed by its inclusion as a demonstration sport at the 1996 Atlanta Paralympic Games, and an official medal sport at the 2000 Sydney Paralympic Games. As of June 2022, a total of 35 countries have wheelchair rugby world rankings, with the sport dominated by Japan, Great Britain, the US, and Australia.

What rules, if any, does it have?

To make wheelchair rugby a fair sport, the IWRF developed an athlete classification system to ensure teams are evenly matched. The system assigns points and half points to all players (0.5 up to 3.5) based on their level of functional movement, with the lowest scores given to players with the least amount of movement. These point allocations are important for team selection and game substitutions because a team can only have four players on the court at a time, and their total athlete score cannot exceed eight points. This ensures diversity and inclusion, because teams are unable to overly rely on athletes with good functioning in their upper bodies. Other basic rules include:

- The ball must be bounced or passed every 10 seconds
- After inbounding the ball, the attacking team have 12 seconds to progress the ball over the halfway line, and 40 seconds to score
- Attacking players cannot linger in the opposition's defensive zone, or 'key', for more than 10 seconds, and defending players cannot have more than three players in the key at any one time
- For player safety reasons, chairs cannot be struck behind the axle of the rear wheel

The joy of it all

Richard (Dickie) is 31 years old and a current member of the Australian Steelers wheelchair rugby team. He also works for Paralympics Australia in a voluntary game-development role. He loves this job, because it allows him to give back to a sport that's been super important in his life, a sport that gave him a strong sense of purpose after a freak accident changed his life.

When Dickie was 19, he was swimming in a pool at a friend's house. Everyone was having a great time, that is, until a mate tried to jump over him, misjudged, and kneed Dickie in the back of the head. The impact crushed his neck and immediately paralysed him. He was rushed to hospital where he commenced a two-month spinal injury rehabilitation, with several operations, following by a further six months of in-patient rehabilitation. For Dickie, who had played soccer and rugby union at school, it was the cruellest of fates.

Ready to get back into life

According to Dickie, when you suffer an injury like his, it takes about two years to recover enough from the shock, the multiple operations, and the rehabilitation before you can genuinely re-engage with life. In time, he got more and more frustrated with missing out on things, so he started going to the gym three times a week, and when a friend suggested he try wheelchair rugby, he was eager to give it a go. He'd seen the sport on TV, but he didn't know much about it. So, he went along to a give-it-a-go day, put on some gloves, got in a chair, and started pushing. Almost immediately, something clicked in his mind and body. This was something he could do! It was a sport that, metaphorically speaking, levelled the playing field by adjusting for different levels of physical impairment. Despite limited movement in his arms, and an inability to grip, Dickie was able to get involved. And get involved he did!

According to the IWRF classification system, Dickie is a 1.5 athlete, which makes him a defensive player, with primary responsibilities for blocking attacking players, and because of his limitations with catching and passing the ball, an occasional ball handler. But just knowing there was a role for him made a difference. It gave him a sense of purpose and fired up some ambition. It was just the thing he needed.

Murder ball and 'killin' it' in life!

Wheelchair rugby can be a difficult sport to get started in, difficult because everybody who comes to the sport is different – different degrees of limb function and trunk stability, and different body sizes and shapes. This means that the wheelchairs used must be custom made to suit the unique specifications of each athlete. And then there are the physical demands of pushing a chair and the skill of manoeuvring it, along with playing a contact sport and understanding game strategy. For Dickie, these were just problems to be solved, and after all he had been through, good ones to be facing.

In his first 12 months of wheelchair rugby, Dickie accomplished a lot. As an athlete, he solved some of the initial problems mentioned above and started training three times a week, with an additional two sessions in the gym. As a result, his physical strength increased significantly and his game improved. It led him to complete his first competition in Melbourne and be selected to play for his state. Not bad for his first year.

Perhaps more importantly, as a person, Dickie found himself becoming more independent. The strength he'd developed in wheelchair rugby allowed him to start living without the help of his carers. But this independence was also inspired by his teammates, by what he saw them do during their interstate trips, and how they dealt with their everyday challenges. Dickie discovered that rugby was about so much more than rugby. His confidence skyrocketed, as did his satisfaction with life.

More highs, more lows, and more highs again

In 2014, Dickie made the Australian team, a real highlight for him and something that would lead to more amazing experiences. He was training with the national squad, travelling to international tournaments, and making friends all over the world. But it all felt a bit surreal, a bit like he needed a pinch to make sure it was happening.

Then life gave him one hell of a pinch. It started when he lost his place on the national team in 2015. Whilst he kept playing and stayed committed, in 2016 the pinch turned into a punch. He was diagnosed with an autoimmune disease, myasthenia gravis, that left him with double vision and barely able to open his eyes or move his arms. This had no connection to his original injury, but it landed him back in hospital again – this time for two months – with a medical treatment plan that included immune suppressant medication and regular plasma exchange to 'clean' his blood.

Undeterred, Dickie knew he'd come too far to let this stop him. By 2018, although still not fully recovered, he was back in the national team and made several trips to tournaments in the US and UK. Along the way, he had another operation to remove his thymus to try to improve his immune responses. This led to a further overhaul of his medication regime and a lifelong dependence on it. But, still, he kept going, He had his eyes on a big prize: the 2021 Tokyo Paralympic Games.

Toyko, Paris and all the other good things

Dickie did indeed make it to Tokyo. Like so many athletes, this was the realisation of a dream. Even though he only got on court for a couple of minutes throughout the tournament, just being there was a thrill. And why wouldn't it be? He had got there despite multiple setbacks, and was able to train with the team and find various ways to make himself useful. Sure, COVID-19 restrictions stripped the event of its opening and closing ceremonies, and its crowds, but the venues were impressive, and the media still wanted to interview him! As far as he was concerned, given what he had been through to get there, that was enough. After all, there's always Paris 2024…

You could excuse Dickie, were he to look back on the past 12 years and feel a bit cheated by life. Cut down in his prime, challenged by life in a wheelchair, only to have his immune system compromised. But whilst that's more than anyone should have to deal with, Dickie doesn't think he's been cheated. Rather than looking back, he looks forward, looking for further things he can create and achieve. Wheelchair rugby has made that easier.

It's given him a game he enjoys playing. When he's on the court, his disability fades away. He likes the strategy of it – the way teams rotate their players, force turnovers, and manage their defensive and offensive time limits. Then, there's the intensity of it. The collisions and the noise, the off-the-ball play. Wheelchair rugby is highly dynamic, and no place for the faint of heart.

It's also a game that changes lives. It sure changed his. Not only did it allow him to travel the world, but he also met his fiancée through rugby, and it has presented him with a great opportunity to help others. As a result of all that, he's become a confident person with a real sense of purpose, a purpose that's about sharing the sport with others: going to spinal rehabilitation units, working his networks, and doing whatever he can to support others dealt a rough hand by life. Offering them hope and a way forward through a special, albeit rather rugged, sport.

X (Cross) Country Running

What is it?

As far as physical pursuits are concerned, running is the purest of the lot. Pure in the sense that running is fundamental to our make-up, so much so that some say human beings are 'born to run'. Physiologically and biomechanically, there's plenty of evidence to back up that statement, especially when running long distances. For one thing, we sweat when we run, which keeps our body temperature within good working limits. In contrast, animals don't sweat. Instead, when they run, they quickly overheat and must stop to cool down. From an evolutionary perspective, this has given humans a massive advantage. If you need any convincing, search up 'persistence hunting' on the internet. You'll soon appreciate the importance of running to our species.

As a specific form of sport and recreation, running comes in many forms. It can occur over a variety of distances, whether it's 100-metre sprints or 200-mile ultramarathons, and over a variety of terrains (road, track, or cross-country tracks and trails). As a result, the training programs of competitive and recreational runners vary widely, depending on their preferred distance and terrain. As the title suggests, this chapter focuses on running longer distances and across natural terrain. It's the sort of running that happens across country, and has gained popularity precisely because people can compete or just do it for fun. (And where occasionally down-shifting to a fast hike is an entirely respectable choice.)

What are its origins?

It's a bit of a stretch to determine when and where running originated. What are we going to say? Running started hundreds of thousands of years ago on an African savannah? Certainly, if you asked that question about tennis or golf, you'd get a more definitive answer. Why? Because they aren't naturally evolved forms of human movement but were invented by someone at some time, primarily as a form of entertainment. But running isn't like that. Along with walking, it's our most natural form of movement.

What about the origins of running for recreational and sporting purposes? For that, ancient Greece isn't a bad place to go in search of answers. Records of competitive running appear as far back as the first Olympic Games (776 BC), and in the writings of the philosopher Plato. It's also possible that competitive running commenced in Ireland, many centuries earlier, at funeral events called the Tailteann Games. Whatever way you come at the question of its origins, you are left with the basic conclusion that organised running has been around for a very long time. Rather than split hairs about exactly when and where it got started, let's agree that the modern Olympic Games played a fairly important role in popularising the sport.

What rules, if any, does it have?

It also seems a little odd to dwell on the rules of running. As a form of human movement, running doesn't have rules per se. Sure, there's good technique and poor technique, but no rules as such. That means people can run and jog recreationally without thinking too much about it. Rules only become relevant when people start competing, including when they run off-road. But even then, running doesn't have rules about *how* someone runs. That only happens in race walking, where athletes must always have one foot touching the ground. There are no such rules in any of the running disciplines. People can run in whatever way they like. And they do. There is arguably nothing more diverse in this world as individual running styles.

The rules in X (cross) country running relate more to when and where people run. For example, most ultramarathons trail runs these days have set cut-off times about either finishing the race or passing through set checkpoints on course. That helps to control when people run, but the primary rules govern where people run. Regardless of the distance of a X (cross) country running event, it always follows a set course. If you stray from the course, disqualification awaits.

The joy of it all

Melissa is a 40-year-old software developer. She's also an avid beekeeper in her spare time, and a more than avid trail runner. In fact, she's an amazing trail runner, the sort that leaves you a bit speechless. Need an example? In April 2022, Melissa ran an event called Irrational S.O U.T.H., a 200-mile event held near Adelaide, in South Australia. After running for just over 62 hours (and sleeping for a total of about an hour), Melissa crossed the line at 9.03 p.m. on a Friday night. She finished in first place, nearly two hours ahead of the first male, and nearly three hours ahead of the second-placed female. Clearly, a remarkable feat of endurance.

Now, you'd understand it then if she had taken herself off to bed for a well-earned rest and a nice sleep-in. As it happened, she did the first part, but not the second. She fell into bed that night, having informed her support crew (her mum) that she was setting an alarm for 7 a.m. Her plan? To get up and run 5 km in the local parkrun mere hours after running roughly 350 kilometres over three days. Remarkably, she did get up, and she did do it. Even more remarkably, she completed the course in under 25 minutes. That's a highly respectable time by any standards. And guess what? That's not even the first time she's pulled that stunt.

She did something similar after a comparable 2019 event in Western Australia.

Clearly, Melissa loves to run, and she's very good at it. Those who know her stand back and marvel at what she achieves. But Melissa is more nonchalant. Down-to-earth and humble, she says she just enjoys the challenges she takes on, and that her training habits prepare her well for all of them, so whenever she conquers a challenge, it's a relatively low-key affair. She seems to treat it as a trigger to start focusing on the next thing, whilst anyone else is still trying to make sense of what she's done.

Life before trail running

Melissa wasn't always a runner. As a kid she played netball and, a bit later, softball. However, although she quite enjoyed the competitive side of those sports, she didn't take them too seriously. Melissa was also involved in karate for many years, which she liked but wasn't terribly adept at. Meanwhile, during her childhood and adolescence, Melissa's parents were living an adventurous lifestyle. This meant she spent lots of time in and around national parks, travelling the state, exploring landscapes, and indulging her mum's great passion: bushwalking, or 'forced marches' as the family came to affectionately call them.

As a result of all this outdoor exposure, Melissa became very comfortable with being in nature, although, up to that point, she'd had no urge to run through it. That all changed in her mid-twenties, when she moved to Sydney and started doing some 20-minute runs around a local park. Then, when some friends decided train for the annual City-to-Surf 14-km fun run, she started running in a group for the first time. This was also her first experience of following any sort of training plan, which she quite liked. In time, she would realise that race planning was something she had quite a talent for.

A fusion of interests

Having found road running, it was inevitable that, at some point, she'd take it off-road. And she did. She did some of the obstacle races quite popular at the time, events like Tough Mudder that were more adventurous than road running and resulted in you getting your feet wet and your face muddied. This greatly increased the fun factor for her and, lo and behold, she quickly started winning events. Not only did she have some talent for it, she also had the right amount of determination and competitive drive. Unfortunately, the expansion of obstacle races came with several rule changes – obstacles became higher and weights became heavier. As Melissa is slightly built, and not blessed with great height, these changes were more of a struggle for her. She not only found it harder to win events, she also found it harder to complete them. After all, when you're five feet three inches tall, getting over an eight-foot high barrier is near on impossible. It was time to look for something else.

At this point, Melissa got inspired by her dad. He'd been a runner for years and become keen on trail running. This included a completion of the legendary 46-km Six-Foot Track ultramarathon in the Blue Mountains, west of Sydney. Taking her cues from this, Melissa decided to give it a go too. The Six-Foot Track was her first foray into longer distance events, and by training for it, she blended several interests into one: her love of green space, outdoor adventuring, a decent challenge, and competition. For Melissa, it was a mix that was always going to work.

Curiouser and curiouser

Of all the things Melissa enjoys about X (cross) country running, the adventure component is probably the greatest. Unlike road running, trail running courses aren't always clearly marked out, especially in the very long distance events. This means you must be able to read a map, or at least follow course instructions. It also means doing this in the dark, although that's a challenge she really likes. Running trails also takes her to interesting places she's never been before. Given she's an innately curious person, that's cool too. Sometimes, during a race, her curiosity will get triggered by an interesting cave, hilltop, or branch of a river. And although she's unable to stop, because she's racing, she'll make a mental note and, if possible, go back for a closer look on another day. As a result, Melissa has become a walking guidebook of the many trails, caves, rivers, coastal strips, and mountains of the NSW Central Coast.

Then there's the competitive side of the sport. That's something she enjoys, whether she's running 5 km on an athletics track or 100 km on a trail. But the running is only one part of the competitive experience. She also enjoys the planning and logistical side of her longer races: planning rest stops, nutrition packs, her pacing strategy for a race, etc. Everything, that is, except sleep breaks, which is a much more see-how-you-go affair. As every minute sleeping is a minute not competing, Melissa tries to keep it to a minimum. But because the body insists on what the body needs, if she ever starts hallucinating or stumbling (falling asleep whilst running), she'll lie down for a micro nap.

Fresh Hell

Yet another thing Melissa loves about running is the social side of the sport. Admittedly, running often involves time spent alone, but much of Melissa's training happens in some sort of group, one organised by others or herself, like the 5 a.m. 'Fresh Hell' hill training group that Melissa leads once a week in a local forest. This enthusiastic group of nutters enjoys the challenge of a steep hill, whilst sharing Melissa's passion for using foot power to explore the world. They, like many running groups, are a positive and supportive team that provide a steady stream of good-natured banter and encouragement to all, through good times and bad.

Surprisingly, Melissa can imagine her life without this type of running. The way she figures it, she'll probably be competitive for another 10 years, after which time she'll likely transition to orienteering or regaining. Whatever she does, she'll be in there competing, doing things at a slower pace but keeping an even closer eye on potential places for future adventuring.

Yachting

What is it?

Like kayaking, alpine skiing, and surfing, the term yachting is rather broad, but most commonly it refers to the competitive and recreational use of boats powered by wind and sails. As such, it includes sailing vessels that vary significantly in size, from small one-person dinghies to much larger ocean-going 'super-maxis'. Strictly speaking, it can also include other forms of watercraft powered only by wind, such as windsurfers, kitesurfers, and even model sailboats, but this is not what people generally associate with the term.

Yachting is a form of sport and recreation with true international appeal, especially for people who live in island nations and countries that border an ocean or sea. Due to the variability in sailboats, people interested in the sport have lots of options about how and where they might sail. In addition, the sport provides good options for learners (with many starting in small single-sail dinghies) and people of varying age and physical capability. Having said that, sailing can be quite expensive and involves an array of costs related to mooring fees (for yacht owners) or boat hire (for non-owners), along with equipment, maintenance, and/or race fees. As such, personal financial resources may be a barrier to participation for some people.

What are its origins?

Yachting is yet another form of sport and recreation with ancient origins. The earliest record of a ship being under sail dates back to ancient Egypt, ca. 3500 BC. In terms of transport, few things have wielded a greater impact on world history than the sailboat. Exploited most effectively by numerous European countries during the Age of Exploration (15th–17th centuries), a mastery of sailing was also achieved in the Americas, Asia, the Middle East, Africa, and Polynesia.

The term 'yacht' is often thought to derive from the Dutch word *jaght*, which is 'a swift light vessel of war, commerce, or pleasure'. Clearly, the third meaning is of most interest here. Formal yacht racing is thought to have started in the 17th century, in both Holland and Britain, where (in 1661) King Charles II of England was involved in a race between two royal sailing vessels. By the 19th century, recreational sailing had increased in popularity so much that the first yacht clubs in European and North America were established. In 1851, the New York Yacht Club and the Royal Yacht Squadron met for the first time to contest the America's Cup, and by 1896, sailing had become so widespread that it was included in the first modern Olympic Games in Athens. Yachting, or sailing as it is now known, has featured in every Games since that time, with the exception of the 1904 St Louis Olympics.

What rules, if any, does it have?

The rules surrounding yachting are many and varied. In competitive situations, the basic aim of yacht racing is to complete a set course in the shortest possible time. When racing in regattas, winners are decided after several races, with points accumulated in each race according to each boat's finishing position. Beyond that, there are rules to govern how boats are equipped and crewed, how they start races, how they communicate, how they proceed around a designated course, and how penalties are enforced for rule infringements.

Race rules differ according to yacht class, with an overarching set of universal rules that stipulate what boats should and should not do on the water, regardless of whether they are competing or not. Many rules relate to safety, primarily avoiding contact between boats on the water, such as stipulating when boats must give way to others, and how they should change direction to avoid collisions.

The joy of it all

Emma is a very busy 21-year-old. She a full-time athlete, a business owner, and a part-time exercise science student. She started sailing at the age of seven, when her older sister took her to a Bring-a-Friend Day at a local sailing club. Eager to keep up with whatever her big sister did, she was excited to go. That all changed a few hours later, when she was pushed out onto Sydney Harbour in a wooden sailing dinghy. She quickly went from excited to petrified, and cried her way through the whole experience.

Therefore, it would be stretching the truth to claim that Emma loved sailing right from the start. It's hard to love something that scares you silly. But it didn't take too long before she experienced some mixed feelings – liking it a bit, despite her tears. It was when she started sailing with a good friend that things really started to change. She distinctly remembers sailing a dinghy with a smiley face painted on its deck. This helped to change her perspective and see that if other people enjoyed sailing, she might too. It was a key moment, a moment that (if you'll pardon the pun) hoisted the sail on her love affair with the sport.

Like going to school without the grades

By the time Emma was 11, sailing had become a big part of her life. She'd become good enough to compete, and was racing almost every weekend. She raced so much that the sailing club became her second home. She'd arrive early on a Saturday morning, pair up with another junior sailor, go out and race, come back in for lunch, pair up with someone else, and go out to do it all over again, that afternoon. At the end of the day, her family would have dinner at the club, so she'd stay for a while before going home to sleep, and come back on Sunday to repeat the process.

At that time in her life, the sailing club was an incredibly positive place to be. Emma was learning how to be a sailor and how to race, and doing so in a big cohort of kids. They spent a lot of time with each other, acquiring key knowledge and skills, like how to do boat checks, organise rigging, get in and out of wetsuits, and more. And because the older kids would help the younger kids, it was like going to school without being segregated by age grades. They were a group of young people having a great time, whilst becoming responsible enough to sail a yacht safely.

From skiffs to Nacra

It turned out that Emma had quite a talent for sailing. She spent the next few years working her way through the various youth classes, as a 'skiffy'. That means she was sailing small single-hulled skiffs, which she raced in until she was 15. By then, some good things were starting to happen. Emma was awarded a sailing scholarship, started to represent her state, and transitioned into sailing Olympic-class yachts. This was where the fun really started, because that meant catamarans and speed!

By the time Emma was 18, she had progressed to the Nacra15 junior boat and, soon after, the Nacra17. What, you might wonder, is a Nacra? It's a fair question. A Nacra is a foiling catamaran. This means the yacht has two hulls, with two hydrofoils attached to each hull, situating the boat higher in the water than other models; sometimes it sits above the water, because the foils create lift. As a result, the boats go much faster, because there is less boat in the water to create drag. Sailing like this is something that Emma really likes.

Fast and technical

The design of a Nacra makes these boats highly manoeuvrable. When you add speed to the equation, you've got a yacht that can be quite a handful. So, you need to know what you're doing, as if you don't have the right level of experience and skill, you could easily get hurt. This makes Nacra sailing highly technical and presents challenges that Emma enjoys. If she had to choose her favourite from all the different yacht classes she's sailed, she says, it would be a Nacra17. For her, it's no contest. Why? A few reasons.

First, Emma doesn't like sailing alone. She likes a good chat and partnering with others. In the Nacra class, boat crews are mixed, with one female and one male on board. Second, she's found that a Nacra provides a good return for effort, which is not true of all boats. That means effort on the boat is directly proportional to the speed achieved on the water – the more effort you put in, the faster you go. This brings us to the third reason: Emma loves going fast, and so she finds Nacra racing exciting and completely absorbing. To do it well, she has to be fully focused on what she's doing, totally synchronised with her partner, fearless, fast, and strong. This leads us nicely to another aspect of sailing she loves – the training.

'She's a beast!'

At five feet five inches tall, Emma is shorter than most female sailors her age. As she climbs towards the top of the sport, the feedback is always the same: 'You need to get heavier; you need to get stronger'. Understanding the importance of the advice, and not wanting it to impede her progress, Emma has accepted the feedback and done something about it. As it happens, she's done quite a lot about it.

Keen to act on the advice, 16-year-old Emma decided to give CrossFit a go. It turned out to be a great choice, because the intensity of CrossFit training aligned well with the reality of Nacra17 sailing. She went looking for the two things female sailors need to develop the most, grip strength and upper body strength, and that's precisely what she got. How could she not, when she was doing dozens of legless rope climbs, push-ups, pull-ups, and walking handstands? But it wasn't just helping her upper body strength; her lower body strength was also improving, as was her confidence. As she described it, being able to do 100 squats, or 100 of anything, was a revelation for her. She was gaining confidence in her physical capacity in the gym, and it was translating to her life on the boat.

Best of all, she loves the gym environment. Not only has it allowed her to (quite literally) address her weaknesses, but it also gave her something else to compete at, like the CrossFit Games. This made it fun and exciting. The strength and speed she has developed, too, has become a point of difference for her, and a competitive advantage on the water. It's something that's been captured on social media and spread through word-of-mouth, the reputation that, whilst she might be a bit smaller than most, Emma's 'a beast!'

Life without sailing? Yeah, right!!

It's hard for Emma to imagine a life without sailing. Like, really hard. It's been such a part of her life. She's lived it since she was seven years old and now, close to the top of the sport, she's totally focused on some very big goals. Naturally, that involves the Olympics: Paris (2024), Los Angeles (2028), and hopefully Brisbane (2032). As such, she's not stopping anytime soon. Any why would she? Sailing is well and truly in Emma's blood. It has given her so much enjoyment and satisfaction, has provided lifelong friendships, allows her to see the world, and has taught her a lot about herself and what she's capable of doing. Importantly, it's also given her a way to promote the sport, by sharing with others how working hard off the water really helps to support success on the water.

Zurkhaneh

What is it?

Zurkhaneh means more than one thing. Translated from Persian, it means 'House of Power' or 'House of Strength'. As such, it refers to a specific type of building, a gymnasium of sorts, where people – mostly men – engage in strength and conditioning training that combines Persian yoga, calisthenics, and aerobic and resistance exercises. Collectively, the exercises are referred to as zurkhaneh arts or sports. As such, this chapter will simultaneously refer to a physical location (the zurkhaneh) and seven disciplines performed within it. The disciplines are based on martial exercises that have been used to train Iranian warriors for thousands of years. They include the *meel* (the swinging of clubs), *kabadeh* (the chained bow), *sang* (exercise with shields), *shena* (push-ups), *charkh* and *pazadan* (whirling and cardio-aerobic exercise), and *koshti pahelvani* (which preceded freestyle wrestling). This makes training sessions a systematic re-enactment of an ancient style of battle done in a symbolic way.

A zurkhaneh is somewhat like a gym, but in many ways it is not the same. This is most obvious when entering a zurkhaneh, where the entrance is set lower than a typical doorway to ensure athletes bow in an act of humility before God and each other. In addition, sessions are led by a respected community leader (*morshed*, or master) who sits above a circular workout pit (*gowd*) and recites moral poetry whilst beating a drum (*zarb*). These aspects of zurkhaneh carry considerable cultural and religious significance, making it strongly wholistic.

What are its origins?

The roots of zurkhaneh can be traced back over thousands of years to the training protocols used by Persian armies, which aimed to develop the physical, mental, and moral strength of warriors. Whilst the geo-political history of the Persian region has seen zurkhaneh fall in and out of favour over the centuries, the practice has steadfastly endured. This appears to be, in large part, because of its symbolism and standing as a source of Iranian pride and deep culture. An important part of this is its underpinning morality – akin to a code of chivalry – where the development of athleticism was prized not only a means of national defence but also as a way of enabling one to redeem the rights of the helpless and poor from their oppressors.

Clearly, this brief origin statement fails to capture the richness and texture of zurkhaneh, so we will simply say that it originated during the time of the Persian empire, is still widely practiced in Iran, and since the International Zurkhaneh Sport Federation was established in 2004, has been promoted in over 70 countries. Interestingly, most of the Iranian wrestling team are zurkhaneh practitioners, something that is often cited as a reason for Iran's prominence in that sport for over 50 years. Of the 76 Olympic medals won by Iran at various Summer Olympic Games, 47 have been in wrestling.

What rules, if any, does it have?

Given that zurkhaneh is not a competitive sport, there are no rules to list as such. Rather, there are certain requirements that athletes are expected to adhere to:

- New athletes to the zurkhaneh are not permitted to train immediately; rather, they must sit and observe the rituals and practices of the zurkhaneh for several weeks before they are allowed to participate

- In line with its underpinning morality, athletes are expected to be pure, truthful, and good tempered, as these are considered pre-requisites for being strong in body
- The hierarchy within a zurkhaneh is based on training age, not chronological age; athletes are expected to show respect to athletes who possess more experience than they do, irrespective of age, social status, or physical strength

The joy of it all

Dr Kashi Azad is a 44-year-old entrepreneur who runs a Persian yoga and chiropractic business. Prior to becoming a professional practitioner, he was an electrical engineer and ran a technology business for several years. Although successful, he did not find it fulfilling. Kashi, however, was very interested in bodywork and physical conditioning, which he pursued through competitive mixed martial arts and during his 18 years as a boxing trainer. Although he had some awareness of zurkhaneh through his cultural heritage, it wasn't until 2007, when he was in his mid-twenties, that he first experienced it. After receiving an invitation to train, Kashi went along, confident that his mixed martial arts experience meant he was well equipped. He could not have been more wrong.

Sometimes life surprises you

There were two things that impressed Kashi about that first visit. One was how much the session challenged him. Despite having undergone years of focused physical training, he was surprised to find his strength endurance tested so substantially. The other was how astonished he was by how strong many of the older athletes were. As Kashi struggled through his first workout, he was surrounded by athletes in their forties and fifties who displayed outstanding physical condition and coped well with the seven disciplines. This was evident from the start of the session, when he confronted the first discipline, push-ups with the shena board. This proved much harder than he had anticipated, and he found himself struggling to do 50, whereas the older men easily exceeded this, most performing close to 200 push-ups without so much as a pause.

Kashi's first visit to a zurkhaneh was a 'Eureka!' moment. He'd done years of diligent training for his mixed martial arts, but he'd never experienced anything like this. He found the sight of these older men going about their training, with such discipline and moving with such grace, to be very profound. Although he wasn't conscious of it at the time, it was just what he'd been looking for. A way to develop ageless strength, and age gracefully. A systematic approach with a symbolic beauty that strongly resonated for him and, better still, appeared to be highly effective.

With that, Kashi's life changed. He started attending regularly, and so began his first year as a zurkhaneh practitioner.

Traditional arts for a modern world

In the 15 years since his first visit, Kashi's commitment to the philosophy, spirituality, and cultural aspects of zurkhaneh has only increased. Indeed, today his business is dedicated to raising awareness about the zurkhaneh arts, which includes using his training studio to introduce people to the seven disciplines. Somewhat controversially, he has welcomed women to the practice and been criticised as a result. Why? Because, in Iran, zurkhaneh is undertaken exclusively by men. The belief amongst traditionalists is that the arts should only be performed by men, the result of religious doctrine that was introduced after the Arab Muslim conquest of Persia.

Nonetheless, Kashi made the decision to include women for two reasons. The first was a simple business decision. By allowing women to train, he substantially increased his target market. He also felt uncomfortable denying anyone the right to train in that way, if they wanted to. 'Who am I to say no?' he points out. The second reason reflects his desire to be an enabler of healthy ageing for others. He derives a strong sense of purpose from openly sharing the benefits of the zurkhaneh arts and wants to do it with the whole world, not just half the world. He notes that whilst zurkhaneh was invented by men, for men, and traditionally focused on the development of masculinity, there is nothing about any of the arts that is beyond the capability of women. This is particularly true, considering that boys often start training at the early age of seven, with exercises regressed and progressed to match the capabilities of each athlete (such as the use of smaller and lighter meels). As far as Kashi is concerned, there is no physical reason to exclude women from practicing these arts. Sure, the disciplines are challenging, and women will be challenged by them – but they are challenging for everyone. That's the whole point.

Not linear but circular

So, what's the joy of it all, according to Kashi? Well, that's not an easy question to answer because a commitment to the zurkhaneh arts is very wholistic, with a spirituality bound to a belief that people can attain truth from the development of strength, truths about oneself and one's existence. No distinction is made between the physical and spiritual body. So, although the self-insights to emerge from practicing zurkhaneh may be similar to those gained through a commitment to running, skiing, or surfing, the distinct difference is that the practice of zurkhaneh follows a structured and systematic process, underpinned by a clear philosophy.

Related to his passion for this is Kashi's deep appreciation of systems. With his engineering background, he knows that a system is designed to maximise efficiency and results. He sees this in zurkhaneh: a body movement system that treats the body as a system, a musculoskeletal system designed to move in a smooth and coordinated way, which is what the seven disciplines aim to do. But this is very different to what happens in a western gym. In most gyms, the approach is to isolate specific muscles and joints, and work them one at a time in a set sequence, e.g., upper body on Mondays, lower body on Wednesdays, and core exercises on Saturdays.

This linear approach to body work is something Kashi struggles with, even though it's the approach he used as a mixed martial artist. These days, he says, it makes little sense to him. The circularity of zurkhaneh makes better sense, as it symbolises the continuous, fluid nature of human strength and conditioning. But circularity is more than just a symbol. It is seen everywhere in the Zurkhane. For example, the main training area – the gowd – is circular. It organises athletes into a circle, around which they perform many circular movements, like meel swinging and whirling, that are designed to hone the human body as a whole, without segmenting it.

Be tireless!

There are many things that Kashi values about zurkhaneh. He likes that it's a simple system that strengthens mind and body, and encourages him to live with passion, energy, humility, and compassion. He likes that it promotes a sense of community and mutual encouragement through the custom of ending sessions by shaking hands and wishing others to 'be tireless', a gesture that really sums up the ethos of zurkhaneh: the encouragement to be young at heart and tireless in life, in strength, in practice, and in the work of becoming who you really are.

All of this prompted me to ask how have his 15 years practice changed him. How has he grown? Kashi pondered this for a few moments. Not because he didn't have an immediate answer; I'm sure he did. Rather, after contemplating this myself, I think it was because such a question could easily lead to hubris, to make a claim about himself that might be overstated or lacking in humility. Such a response would be inconsistent with how Kashi is living his life, which is supported by his practicing of the zurkhaneh arts. Instead, he shared some feedback he often gets from others, that people experience him as embodying the zurkhaneh ethos in a wholehearted way. And he's understandably happy with that. After all, he was attracted to the arts because of a desire to live as well as he could possibly live. And it appears he's doing just that.

Endnote

In putting this book together, we have clearly omitted many physical pursuits that could have been just as easily included. For instance, we could have spent time highlighting the enjoyment that accompanies participation in lawn bowls, trampolining, rogaining, taekwondo, basketball, soccer, badminton, volleyball, any of the athletics field events (high jump, javelin, pole vault, etc.), triathlon, gymnastics, and ice hockey, to name but a few.

For those disappointed at any of these omissions, we hope you aren't too disappointed. This book was always about stimulating expansive thinking about physical activity, summoning your imagination, and tweaking your curiosity such that you might venture forth and try something different. We hope we have achieved that.

But, what about dancing?!

One of the most delightful things about writing a book is hearing from people whose paths you might not otherwise cross. Readers who feel compelled to make contact because of something you've written, and the impact it has had. People like Yvonne.

We first heard from Yvonne quite late in the writing process for this book. We only had a couple of interviews to go, with the table of contents long since defined. Her message came quite out of the blue. We didn't know her, and she didn't know us. But she'd bought a copy of *Get Moving Keep Moving* on a Friday and finished it by the next Monday. It appeared to have had quite a positive impact on her and she was kind enough to share some of that with us. However, she also had a question:

> My big question ... Why does dancing not get a notable mention?
>
> I think adding dancing would round it out a bit better. Especially for the women who danced as girls.

This kicked off a brief exchange of messages. It began with us thanking her for the positive feedback and the suggestion. We continued by informing her that the follow-up book was almost completed, and whilst it highlighted a wide range of physical activity options, dancing had not been included. However, I (GS) did send the following reply:

> To your specific question, although dancing is not covered, I have an ex-student who dances salsa in Queensland & posts the most joyful photos on Facebook. So, I am going to include something of her experience in the final chapter ... you have just sealed that decision (which I had been seriously thinking about)
>
> Many thanks!

Talk about helping to shape a book as it's being written!

As we mentioned in the preface, this book did not set out to be an encyclopædia of physical pursuits. However, something about Yvonne's question really struck a chord. As any anthropologist will tell you, dancing is a significant form of physical activity. In many traditional, non-western societies it is a core cultural activity that can, during festivals and ceremonies, go on for many hours and closely resemble an endurance sport. On that count alone, it was helpful to have her draw our attention to it.

But Yvonne made a broader point that is worth acknowledging. That is, whilst dancing is not typically thought of as a sport, it can be every bit as energetic, physically challenging, and health promoting as the 26 physical pursuits we have outlined. More than that, as she rightly pointed out, it is a significant physical pursuit for the many, many people who enjoyed dancing as youngsters. As such, we felt we needed one last story. It was time to speak to Pierina.

Meet Pierina

Pierina is a 54-year-old high school art teacher and leadership coach. She first started dancing when she was six or seven, when she embarked on a 10-year learning journey focused on ballet, tap, and jazz. This, along with competitive swimming, was something she loved to do. It all made for a busy life, but Pierina loved her activity schedule. However, by the time she turned 16, it was time for a bit of focused high school study, so she paused dancing and swimming to commit more to her academic pursuits.

What happened next? You guessed it. Life. Yes, that's right, life went and got all busy on her. No surprises there – career, relationships, kids, more study. These competing demands conspired to lead Pierina away from some of the things she cared for the most, including dancing, for nearly 30 years.

Reconnecting with a little help from her friends

Pierina found her way back to dancing eight years ago, courtesy of a few life changes and some input from friends. Although her love of dance appeared to have slipped Pierina's mind, this was not the case for her friends. Indeed, it was their comments that helped to reawaken her. Comments like 'You've always been a dancer', and 'If we go anywhere with a dance floor, you are ALWAYS on it!'

With her awareness raised and a little more time on her hands, Pierina decided it was time to reconnect. She chose something she'd always been curious about: Latin dancing. She found a class and, despite feeling a little nervous, went along. Fortunately, Pierina found she wasn't alone. A friend of hers was also taking the class, which made things a bit easier.

However, if Pierina was after an easy option for reconnecting with dance, that's not what she had taken. For one thing, Latin dancing is challenging. The beats, as she says, 'are all over the place', and musically it was completely different to anything she'd ever done before. For another, this was her first experience of partner dancing. All of her childhood ballet, tap, and jazz had been performed solo. So, she had to get used to that intimate element of Latin dance and the relinquishing of control to the lead dancer, her male partner. Having re-engaged with her passion, she still had a lot to learn!

The joy of it all

When Pierina is dancing, she is the very personification of joy. A smile never leaves her face and the enjoyment radiates from her. For her, it is the sheer pleasure of moving to music again, but it is so much more than that.

You see, love of learning is one of Pierina's personal strengths, and Latin dancing has been great for that. She's had to learn about its culture, about its music, and about its movement. She's had to be disciplined and committed to earn the joy she now feels every time she dances. Whilst learning has been an important part, the performance aspects have been another. This became clear to her the first time she performed publicly. She was quickly reminded of how much she loved to perform. How much she enjoyed the build-up – the time spent in the changing room, the surge of adrenaline in the wings, the performance itself, of telling a story and being a character, and then exiting the stage. The whole darn thing!

And when you dance four times a week for two or three hours, you get a solid aerobic and core strength workout – more than enough to satisfy the physical activity recommendations for good health. Dancing does it for Pierina. It keeps her fit, it keeps her strong, and, most importantly, it keeps her happy. So happy that she can't imagine life without dancing, something she intends to do for a very, very long time.

So, thanks to Yvonne, we are happy to declare dancing as Way to Keep Moving #27!

A book of 'one-buttock conversations'

This book has been a joy to write. And why not? When 27 people (26 + Pierina) agree to talk to you about the physical pursuits they love, well, there's a good chance you'll have an enjoyable time. As we found out, that sort of enthusiasm is highly contagious. It's an enthusiasm and passion that can change the way people speak and get them really animated.

It's an energy that creates what we like to call 'one-buttock conversations'. The sort of conversations that elevate people emotionally and get them sitting up in their seats – metaphorically if not physically – on one buttock, eager to share more of their positive experiences.

As a result of all this, we have learnt a great deal. Our horizons have been expanded. Although we felt we possessed a broad knowledge base of different physical pursuits coming into the project, we now know a whole lot more. For example, we've learnt that *goalball* is like doing continuous burpees, that *padel* is an extremely social game, that *quadball* involves plenty of rough and tumble, that *vigoro* is a faster form of cricket, and that *zurkhaneh* is a fascinating blend of physical art form and sport. In addition, we've developed a greater appreciation for the allure of *CrossFit*, the 'communitas' of *dragon boating*, the wackiness of *extreme ironing*, the finesse of *fencing*, the physics of *judo*, the thrill of *luge*, and the spirit of *ultimate*. For everything else, we've been lucky enough to peek behind the curtain at what gives people some of their greatest joy in life. For this we both feel very grateful and privileged. There truly are some wonderfully interesting people in this world!

Social connection: The common thread

As far as the *26 Ways* are concerned, there is something we should point out, and that is the importance that other people play in shaping personal enjoyment of each physical pursuit. As we collected the stories, it became obvious that none of these pursuits would be as good without the social connectivity that comes with them. Fascinatingly, this plays out in myriad ways:

- For Marina, it happens as part of teaching her children how to ski, annual ski trips with family, and sharing her alpine knowledge with others.
- For Neil, it happens as part of a light-hearted annual pilgrimage with some good friends to the side of a bog trench in central Wales.
- For Oliver, it happens as part of the commitment he has to optimising his physical performance, and the safe, supportive environment he creates when coaching others.
- For Donna, it happens as part of being in a boat, paddle in hand, surrounded by enthusiastic, positive people who are committed to living life to the full.
- For Aimee, it happens as part of interacting with her tribe of fun-loving canyoners who extreme iron occasionally.
- For Eddie, it happens as part of his involvement in fencing as a competitor, coach, and organiser, and the expanded social network this has created for him.
- For Tyan, it happened through the synchronisation she had to achieve as a vision-impaired athlete, which infused her sporting relationships with trust and respect.
- For Eleanor, it happens as part of challenging herself on walking tracks and the endlessly interesting and inspiring people she meets.
- For Aylin, it happens as part of trying to master a very challenging, technical sport and being surrounded by likeminded others trying to do the same.
- For Shane, it happens as part of knowing that he can travel the world and turn up, unannounced, to any dojo and be welcomed in for a wrestle.
- For Kesley, it happens both because paddling with others is a basic safety measure and the thrill of surf ski kayaking is therapeutic in a way that creates strong connections.
- For Alex, it happens in being invited to train in teams from bigger, stronger luging nations, and being embraced by the camaraderie that exists within that sport.

- For Vinnie, it happens as part of engaging in the favoured physical pursuits of his childhood with his two teenage boys, which gives it new meaning.
- For Susan, it happens as part of playing her favourite sport with her favourite humans, women she has shared a special netball bond with for up to 25 years.
- For Kristen, it happens at the end of a race, standing on a beach with other swimmers, waiting for the last person to finish and cheering them out of the water.
- For Matt, it happens as part of the festive atmosphere of a padel event, an energising mixture of sport, music, and good food.
- For Alise, it happens as part of playing a sport that is fun and energetic, that values inclusion and welcomes individuals to bring their authentic selves.
- For Zoe, it happens as part of gelling with her crewmates, moving on the water as one, and sharing the special moments that only a sunrise over a lake or river can provide.
- For Kristen, it happens as part of being part of the 'mafia' that is surfing, people who share her passion and have helped to teach her what commitment is really about.
- For Peter, it happens as part of his ongoing recovery from stroke, supported by his deep enjoyment of table tennis, and the care and concern of the people he plays with.
- For Craig, it happens as part of playing a sport that trusts its players to self-referee their matches and interact in a way that maintains a spirit of honesty and fair play.
- For Deanne, it happens as part of continuing a 38-year connection to vigoro and creating a community that supports the physical, mental, and social health of all those who play.
- For Richard, it happens as part of solving his physical challenges in both sport and life, and the inspiration he gets from watching how other wheelchair athletes do it.

- For Melissa, it happens as part of competing in ultra-marathons, supported by friends who run with her at night and listen to her bad singing, whilst they try to keep her sane.
- For Emma, it happens as part of her lifelong connection to an extended sailing family, and the sense of partnership she gets from crewing and racing super swift yachts.
- For Kashi, it happens as part of being involved in a community that shares a rich history, cultural heritage, and shared value in the enhancement of physical and spiritual health.

We hope that we've shown that when we get physically active, there's a whole lot to be said for getting together with others. It's true that social connections tend to come more naturally with team sports, yet only 10 of the physical pursuits in this book can be said to be either a team sport or a physical pursuit undertaken in pairs: dragon boating, goalball, netball, padel, quadball, rowing, ultimate, vigoro, wheelchair rugby, and yachting.

With that in mind, if your interest has been triggered by what strikes you as a solo sport or pursuit, something like open-water swimming, X-country running, or bog snorkelling, know that these options can be as social as you'd like to make them. The opportunities are out there. You just need to find them.

It's time to take enjoyment seriously!

There is one last observation we would like to make. That is, in all the interviews we conducted for this book, and the 27 stories we wrote up, we never got the impression that anyone associated their chosen pursuit with any sense of boredom, drudgery, or personal inconvenience. Rather, everyone reflected on something that they *freely choose to do,* and for some, an activity they simply do not want to be without.

Regrettably, this is not the way many people feel about exercise and physical activity. This is particularly so with the concept of 'exercise', which carries a good deal of baggage for many people.

With that in mind, we advocate for thinking about this in terms of physical activity and physical pursuits. More than that, we advocate for taking enjoyment seriously. So seriously that we believe a reconnection to physical activity is best approached by 'doing some headwork before you do the legwork'. Spend some time thinking about what you're interested in and what you might like, so that you can make one of the best decisions of your life – choosing an enjoyable way to keep moving.

This brings us back to where we started, to this book's predecessor, *Get Moving Keep Moving*, and the Health Activation Process. If you haven't read it yet, or completed the process, now might be a good time to do so. But even if you have read it and completed the process, we suggest you take a quick look back, just in case there's anything worth changing.

Whatever you decide to do, enjoy it!

A note on research and references

The importance of gathering information and other source materials for this book does not rise to the level of most other books. Why? Because this was always primarily a book of personal narratives, captured from 26 (plus 1) interviews. We wanted the stories to be the main players, and needed to provide enough background information to help support the stories.

Nonetheless, we did spend as much time researching each pursuit as we did interviewing, reviewing, and writing up each story. Our research process was straightforward and was conducted mostly online, using a variety of sources. We often began with a Google search for each physical pursuit, which usually led to a relevant Wikipedia page. Knowing that Wikipedia is not always a reliable source of information, we used these pages as convenient starting points and continued our search for information via reference listings and links. More often than not, we found our way to websites and online resources that were administered by an array of national and international governing bodies, sporting associations, recreation clubs, historical societies, and various commercial leisure sites.

In every case, this process yielded enough information for us to: (i) provide a brief description of each physical pursuit, (ii) outline something of its origins, and (iii) make a short statement about its rules, to the extent that each pursuit had formalised rules. By doing this much, we hope we have provided readers with some context to better understand the stories told in each chapter.

The authors

Gordon Spence is an experienced psychologist, educator, researcher, and executive and workplace coach. He holds both a Master's and a PhD degree in coaching psychology from the University of Sydney, along with Bachelor degrees in psychology (University of Wollongong) and exercise and sports science (University of Newcastle). During his 20-year academic career, Gordon has taught a wide variety of subjects, including employee engagement, workplace wellbeing, leadership coaching, and the psychology of peak performance. His scholarly publications include one monograph, two edited books, and over 30 journal articles and book chapters. Gordon is also the author of *Get Moving Keep Moving*, which presents an approach to reconnecting with physical activity via a fusion of psychology and exercise science. A keen runner, Gordon can often be found running on the roads, tracks, or beautiful trails of the NSW Central Coast, where he also coaches novice runners as a qualified recreational run leader.

Riley Spence is a first-time author. He is a Year 10 student who attends Gosford High School and was school captain and dux of Tuggerah Public School. A passionate footballer (soccer), Riley has played since he was four years old, captains the Under 15As team he plays for, and referees local association football. Riley takes a keen interest in a wide range of sports, both as a player (running, basketball, tenpin bowling, table tennis, golf) and a supporter (football, basketball, American football, Australian Football League, rugby league, rugby union, and any Olympic sport, except dressage). Riley also has a part-time job at a local café, has plans to train as a barista prior to leaving school, and pursue further studies in either commerce or exercise science.

Gordon and Riley are father and son. They enjoy running together, are passionate supporters of Liverpool FC and the Parramatta Eels, and share an interest in world history and classic British comedy.

www.ingramcontent.com/pod-product-compliance
Lightning Source LLC
Chambersburg PA
CBHW052011030426
42334CB00029BA/3171